Truly Healthy Meal Ideas
The Natural Ingredients Cooking Guide

Table of Contents

Highland Scotch Egg

Jalapeño Bacon Bites

Fried Green Tomatoes

Bacon Mofongo

Simple Guacamole

Coconut Shrimp

Green Deviled Eggs 'N Ham

Zucchini Rollatini

Healthy Sweets

Frozen Chocolate Cherry Custard

Sugar Cookies

Carrot Cake Cookies

Chocolate Mousse

Banana Bread Pudding

Mixed Berry Trifle

Tapioca Blueberry Crepes

Raw Cocoa Chutney

Red Ants On A Log

Raw Fudge

Raw Banana Cream Pie

Date Butter and Apples
Almond Butter Balls
Red Berry Smoothie
Strawberry Banana Shake
Raw Coconut Chia pudding
Milano Cookie Sandwiches
Berry Tart
Simple Strawberry Cake
Red Velvet Cupcakes
Primal Piña Colada Bars
Sesame Logs
Chocolate Bacon Donut

Health Conscious Baking
Mocha Brownie Bites
Blueberry Scones
Easy Poppy Seed Muffins
Coconut Macaroons
Blackberry Dumplings
Carrot Cake Cookie Bars
Chocolate Zucchini Cak

Cocoa Cream Muffins
Ginger Spice Cookies
Lemon Coconut Bars
Cocoa Spice Pinwheel Cookies
Rosemary Basil Scones
Cinnamon Rolls
Coconut Baked Donut
Blueberry Lavender Blondies
Savory Spiced Pineapple Bread
Strawberry Bread
Apple Cider Bread
No Corn "Corn" Muffins
English Muffins
Easy Pita
Coconut Crisps
Angel Food Cake
Chocolate Mint Milano Cookies

Easy Lunch Recipes
Soft Baked Pita
Cheese Steak Sandwich

Asian Empanada

Turkey Tenders

Soft Baked Pretzel

Frontier Anzac Biscuits

Raw Cashew Avocado Hummus

Zucchini Salad with Sundried Tomato Sauce

Spicy Tuna Tartare

Spinach Mushroom Muffins

Pigs In A Blanket

Mighty Beef Sliders

Quick Chili

Simple Gazpacho + Tortilla Chips

Sweet Potato Fries + Ketchup

Sausage And Peppers Sub

Tuna Sandwich

Kelp Noodle Stir-Fry

Shrimp Taco

Spicy Mango Fried Rice

Seared Tuna Salad

Delectable Dinner Ideas
Parchment Baked Salmon
Smoked Salmon Eggs Benedict
Steak Tartar with Truffle Tapenade
Kelp Noodle Salad with Crunchy Cashew
Sauce
Quick Raw Avocado Slaw
Mango Ginger Apple Salad
Chicken Fries with Garlic Aioli
Chicken Noodle Soup
Cheese Steak Sandwich
Mint Melon Salad
Shrimp Stuffed Squid
Veggie Burger
Crisp Spinach Salad
Chicken Pot Pie
Lamb Pot Pie
Meatballs
Jamaican Jerk Patty
Chicken Tenders
Pizza Bites

Peppercorn Crusted Filet Mignon
Orange Glazed Duck Breast
Clams Casino
Jalapeño Lime Soft Pretzel
Bacon Quesadilla
Chicken Taquitos

Awesome Healthy Pastries
Sweet Potato Pecan Chess Pie
Cocoa-nut Cake
Chocolate Pecan Shortbread Cookies
Peach Pecan "Fried" Pie
Sweet Potato "Fried" Pie
Sugar-Free Coconut Cake
Coconut Cream Pie
Wild Mince Meat Pie
Chocolate Almond Biscotti
Crab Boil Biscuits
Crispy Almond Pizza Crust
Chewy Coconut Pizza Dough
Cashew Belgian Waffles

Double Pumpkin Muffins

Classic Bagels

Plain Pita

Sesame Pretzel Sticks

Chicken Dumpling Bun

Sweet Potato Cinnamon Rolls

Pumpkin Spice Cakes

Fruit And Nut Cake

Toasted Almond Cream Cakes

Healthy Snacks

Cashew Butter And Banana Sandwich

Prep Time: 10 minutes

Cook Time: 20 minutes

Servings: 4

INGREDIENTS

Sandwich Bread

1 cup tapioca flour/starch

1/4 - 1/3 cup coconut flour

1 egg

1/2 cup warm water

1/4 cup coconut oil

1/4 cup applesauce

1 tablespoon sweetener*

1 teaspoon apple cider vinegar

1/2 teaspoon baking soda

1/2 teaspoon cinnamon

1/2 teaspoon sea salt

Filling

1/2 cup cashews (raw or roasted)

2 tablespoons coconut oil

1 tablespoon sweetener*

1/4 teaspoon cinnamon

1 banana

INSTRUCTIONS

1. Preheat oven to 350 degrees F. Line sheet pan with parchment paper or coat with coconut oil.

2. In medium bowl, sift together tapioca flour, 1/4 cup coconut flour, baking soda and salt. Stir in warm water and oil.

3. Whisk egg in small bowl. Add applesauce, vinegar and cinnamon. Add egg mixture to flour mixture and mix until well combined. Add 1 tablespoon coconut flour or water at a time if needed to form soft and slightly sticky dough.

4. Divide dough into 4 portions and roll into round or oval balls. Dust your hand with extra tapioca flour to prevent sticking.

5. Place rolls on sheet pan and pat down slightly. Bake 20 minutes, or until edges are golden brown and the tops are firm. Remove from oven and allow to cool.

6. While *Sandwich Bread* is baking, add cashews, coconut oil, sweetener and cinnamon to food processor or bullet blender and process until smooth. Add 1/2 tablespoon of coconut oil at a time if necessary to reach preferred consistency. Or use jarred cashew butter.

7. Slice bananas. Slice cooled *Sandwich Bread* in half and spread on cashew butter. Layer banana slices on bread.

8. Serve immediately. Or wrap in plastic wrap or parchment and store in lidded container.

*stevia, raw honey or agave nectar

Almond Butter and Strawberry Sandwich

Prep Time: 10 minutes

Cook Time: 20 minutes

Servings: 4

INGREDIENTS

Sandwich Bread

1 cup tapioca flour/starch

1/4 - 1/3 cup coconut flour

1 egg

1/2 cup warm water

1/4 cup coconut oil

1/4 cup applesauce

1 tablespoon sweetener*

1 teaspoon apple cider vinegar

1/2 teaspoon cinnamon

1/4 teaspoon ground ginger

1/2 teaspoon baking soda

1/2 teaspoon sea salt

Filling

1/2 cup almonds (raw or roasted)

2 tablespoons coconut oil

1 tablespoon sweetener*

1/4 teaspoon cinnamon

1/4 teaspoon ground ginger

5 - 6 medium strawberries

INSTRUCTIONS

1. Preheat oven to 350 degrees F. Line sheet pan with parchment paper or coat with coconut oil.
2. In medium bowl, sift together tapioca flour, 1/4 cup coconut flour, baking soda and salt. Stir in warm water and oil.
3. Whisk egg in small bowl. Add applesauce, vinegar, cinnamon and ginger. Add egg mixture to flour mixture and mix until well combined. Add 1 tablespoon coconut flour or water at a time if needed to form soft and slightly sticky dough.
4. Divide dough into 4 portions and roll into round or oval balls. Dust your hand with extra tapioca flour to prevent sticking.
5. Place rolls on sheet pan and pat down slightly. Bake 20 minutes, or until edges are golden brown and the tops are firm. Remove from oven and allow to cool.
6. While *Sandwich Bread* is baking, add almonds, coconut oil, sweetener, cinnamon and ginger to food processor or bullet blender and process until smooth. Add 1/2 tablespoon of coconut oil at a time if necessary to reach preferred consistency. Or use jarred almond butter.
7. Slice strawberries. Slice cooled *Sandwich Bread* in half and spread on almond butter. Layer strawberry slices on bread.
8. Serve immediately. Or wrap in plastic wrap or parchment and store in lidded container.

*stevia, raw honey or agave nectar

Bacon Baked Apples

Prep Time: 15 minutes

Cook Time: 30 minutes

Servings: 4

INGREDIENTS

6 oz nitrate-free bacon (thick slices or whole slab)

4 tart apples

4 dried apricots

2 tablespoons dried cranberries

2 tablespoons dried cherries

2 tablespoons dried raisins

1 tablespoon cinnamon

Juice of half a lemon

Zest of half a lemon

Water

INSTRUCTIONS

1. Preheat oven to 350 degrees F. Heat medium skillet over medium-high heat.
2. Chop apricots. Add dried fruit to small bowl with lemon juice. Add enough water just to cover fruit. Let fruit rehydrate for 10 minutes.
3. Dice bacon and add to hot skillet. Sauté about 5 - 8 minutes, until crisp and golden brown.

4. Slice apples in half lengthwise. Carefully core apples, scooping out seeds, stem and tough core with melon baller. Leave good-sized well in apple.
5. Arrange apples in baking dish just large enough to fit them snuggly. Pour water into bottom of baking dish, about 1/8 inch.
6. Strain fruit, reserving liquid in small bowl. Strain bacon, reserving liquid. Mix lemon zest, cinnamon and bacon with fruit.
7. Fill apple wells with fruit mixture. Press down into apple, packing slightly.
8. Pour 1 teaspoon reserved liquid and over each apple. Follow by 1 tablespoon bacon grease over all 8 apple halves.
9. Bake in preheated oven for 20 - 30 minutes, until apples are tender.
10. Serve warm. Or allow to cooled completely, and store in lidded container.

Sausage And Peppers

Prep Time: 5 minutes

Cook Time: 10 minutes

Servings: 4

INGREDIENTS

4 Italian sausage links (pork, chicken, etc.)

1 white onion

1 bell pepper

INSTRUCTIONS

1. Heat large skillet over medium heat. Add 1 tablespoon coconut oil.
2. Peel onion. Stem and seed pepper. Roughly chop onion and pepper. Slice sausage into 3/4 inch slices.
3. Add sausage to hot oiled skillet and sauté about 2 minutes. Then add onion and peppers. Sauté about 8 minutes, until sausage is cooked through and browned.
4. Serve hot.

Cream Filled Carrot Cake Muffin

Prep Time: 10 minutes*

Cook Time: 20 minutes

Servings: 12

INGREDIENTS

1 1/2 cups almond flour

2 tablespoons tapioca flour

2 eggs

 4 - 6 carrots (1 1/2 cups grated)

1/4 cup coconut oil

1/2 cup unsweetened applesauce

1/4 cup sweetener*

1 teaspoon baking soda

1 teaspoon baking powder

1 tablespoon ground cinnamon

1 teaspoon vanilla

1/2 teaspoon sea salt

Cashew Cream Filling

1 cup cashews

2 - 4 tablespoons sweetener**

1 teaspoon cinnamon

1 1/2 cups water

INSTRUCTIONS

1. *Soak cashews in 1 1/2 cups water overnight. Drain and rinse.

2. Preheat oven to 350 degrees F. Line muffin pan with paper liners or coconut oil.

3. Grate or chop carrot in food processor or bullet blender until coarsely ground. Add to medium mixing bowl with eggs, oil, applesauce and sweetener and beat with hand mixer or whisk.

4. Sift in almond flour, baking soda, baking powder, spices and salt. Mix to combine.

5. Use ice cream scoop or tablespoon to scoop batter into muffin tins 1/2 - 2/3 full.

6. Bake 15 - 18 minutes until muffins are golden brown and tops are firm to the touch.

7. Remove muffins from oven and let cool about 10 minutes.

8. For *Cashew Cream*, process soaked cashews, sweetener and cinnamon in food processor or bullet blender. Add water 1 tablespoon at a time if necessary, just to smooth.

9. Cut hole in top of muffin about 1 inch deep and spoon in *Cashew Cream*. Or fill pastry bag fitted with 1/2 inch tip with Cashew Cream, and inject muffin with cream.

10. Serve warm or room temperature.

**stevia, raw honey or agave nectar*

Baked Sweet Plantains

Prep Time: 5 minutes

Cook Time: 20 minutes

Servings: 1

INGREDIENTS

1 ripe yellow plantain

1 tablespoon sweetener*

2 tablespoons water

1 teaspoon coconut oil

1/2 teaspoon ground cinnamon

INSTRUCTIONS

1. Preheat oven to 400 degrees F. Line baking pan with parchment, or lightly coat with coconut oil.
2. Cut plantain into 3/4 inch slices. Remove peel from each slice.
3. Toss plantains in small bowl with sweetener, water, oil and cinnamon.
4. Arrange plantains in single layer on baking pan. Bake 10 minutes, then turn over and bake another 10 minutes, or until plantains are golden brown and tender.
5. Serve warm.

raw honey or agave nectar

Ants On A Log

Prep Time: 5 minutes

Cook Time: 5 minutes

Servings: 2

INGREDIENTS

3 celery stalks

2 tablespoons raisins

Cashew Butter

1 cup cashews

1 teaspoon coconut oil

1/2 teaspoon ground cinnamon

INSTRUCTIONS

1. Add cashews, cinnamon, and coconut oil to food processor or bullet blender. Process until smooth. Let mixture rest between periods of processing to reach desired consistency, if necessary.
2. Cut celery stakes into thirds and fill wells with *Cashew Butter*. Place raisins on cashew butter.
3. Serve room temperature. Or refrigerate 10 minutes and serve chilled.

Grilled Pineapple Fruit Salad

Prep Time: 5 minutes

Cook Time: 10 minutes

Servings: 4

INGREDIENTS

1/2 pineapple

1 peach

1 cup fresh cherries

1 orange

1 tablespoon fresh mint leaves

Half lemon

INSTRUCTIONS

1. Heat griddle or grill over medium-high heat. Lightly coat with coconut oil.
2. Peel and core pineapple. Cut into half inch slices. Place slice on griddle and grill about 4 - 5 minutes on each side, until grill marks appear and sugars caramelized.
3. Cut peach in half and grill flesh side down for about 5 minutes.
4. Pit cherries and slice in half. Peel orange and cut flesh from white cellulose film and pith.
5. Chop pineapple and peach. Add to medium mixing bowl with cherries and orange wedges. Chiffon mint. Add to bowl and squeeze on lemon juice. Toss to combine.
6. Serve room temperature. Or refrigerate and serve chilled.

Sweet Cinnamon Pretzel

Prep Time: 10 minutes

Cook Time: 20 minutes

Servings: 4

INGREDIENTS

Cinnamon Pretzel

1 cup coconut flour

1/2 cup tapioca flour/starch

1/2 cup coconut oil

1/2 cup water

2 dried dates

1 egg

2 tablespoon apple cider vinegar

1/2 teaspoon baking soda

1/2 teaspoon baking powder

2 teaspoons ground cinnamon

1/2 teaspoon vanilla

1/2 teaspoon ground ginger

1/2 teaspoon sea salt

Coconut Sweet Cream

1/4 cup full-fat coconut milk

2 tablespoons sweetener

1 tablespoon lemon juice

1/2 teaspoon vanilla

INSTRUCTIONS

1. Preheat oven to 350 degrees F. Heat medium pot over medium-high heat. Line sheet pan with parchment or baking mat.

2. Add dates, coconut oil, water, vinegar and salt to food processor or bullet blender and process until smooth. Pour mixture into pot. Bring to a boil and remove from heat.

3. Whisk in tapioca flour. Stir with wooden spoon or soft spatula until mixture gels and comes together.

4. Stir in baking soda and baking powder. Continue mixing for a minute. Mixture will foam and expand. Let mixture sit and cool about 5 minutes.

5. Sift in coconut flour and spices. Mix partially, then beat in egg. Mix until combined. Excess coconut flour may sit in bottom of bowl.

6. Turn out dough onto cutting board dusted with any excess coconut flour from mixture. Knead dough for 2 minutes.

7. Cut dough into 4 equal portions. Roll out pieces into ropes and twist to form classic pretzel twist. Pinch together any crumbled dough.

8. Arrange pretzels on lined sheet pan. Brush with coconut oil or full-fat coconut milk.

9. Place sheet pan in oven and bake about 25 minutes, until cooked through.

10. For *Coconut Sweet Cream*, mix coconut milk, vanilla, sweetener and lemon juice with had mixer or whisk until thick and creamy. Transfer to serving dish.

11. Serve pretzels immediately with *Coconut Sweet Cream*. Or allow pretzels to cool and refrigerate sweet cream, and serve chilled.

stevia, raw honey or agave nectar

Blueberry Dumplings

Prep Time: 15 minutes

Cook Time: 30 minutes

Servings: 6

INGREDIENTS

Blueberry Filling

2.5 cups blueberries (fresh or frozen)

2 - 4 tablespoons sweetener*

2 tablespoons tapioca flour

Dumplings

1/4 cup coconut flour

3/4 cup almond flour

3 tablespoons cold coconut oil

1 teaspoon baking powder

1/2 teaspoon ground cinnamon

1/2 teaspoon ground ginger

1/4 teaspoon sea salt

2 eggs

2 tablespoon sweetener

1 teaspoon vanilla

INSTRUCTIONS

1. Sift coconut flour, almond flour, baking powder and salt into small mixing bowl. Add cinnamon and ginger. Cut in cold coconut oil with fork until crumbly. Place in freezer for 10 minutes.

2. Preheat oven to 400 degrees F.

3. Add blueberries and sweetener to medium pot. Heat over medium heat and bring to simmer. Whisk in tapioca flour and simmer about 10 minutes.

4. Pour blueberries into casserole dish and place in hot oven.

5. In medium bowl, beat eggs, sweetener and vanilla. Add chilled flour mixture to eggs and mix until dough comes together.

6. Carefully remove bubbling blueberries from oven and drop 8 dumplings onto berries.

7. Return dish to oven and bake 15 - 20 min, until dumplings are golden, set and cooked through.

8. Remove dish from oven and allow to cool about 5 minutes.

9. Serve warm. Or allow to cool completely and serve room temperature.

*stevia, raw honey or agave nectar

Papaya Fried Pie

Prep Time: 20 minutes

Cook Time: 20 minutes

Servings: 4

INSTRUCTIONS

Crust

2 cups almond flour

2 eggs

3 tablespoons coconut oil

1 tablespoon sweetener*

1/4 teaspoon baking soda

1/2 teaspoon ground ginger

1/2 teaspoon sea salt

Filling

1 cup papaya (cut into chunks)

1 fresh guava (or 1/2 cup guava puree)

2 tablespoons sweetener*

2 tablespoons water

1 teaspoon vanilla

1/2 inch piece fresh ginger

Zest of half lemon

Juice of half lemon

DIRECTIONS

1. For *Crust*, sift almond flour into medium mixing bowl. Add baking soda, ginger and salt.

2. Whisk eggs and sweetener in small mixing bowl, then add to flour and combine. Slowly add coconut oil until formable dough comes together.

3. Roll in plastic wrap or wrap tightly in parchment and refrigerate for 15 minutes.

4. Preheat oven to 400 degrees. Line sheet pan with parchment or baking mat. Cover cutting board with parchment.

5. For *Filling*, peel, pit and dice papaya. Peel and dice ginger. Add papaya and ginger to food processor or bullet blender with sweetener, water, vanilla, lemon juice and zest, and guava puree, or peeled, seeded guava flesh. Process until smooth.

6. Remove dough from refrigerator. Divide dough into 4 portions. Roll dough into balls and flatten on parchment covered cutting board with hands. Roll into circles about 1/8 inch thick with rolling pin.

7. Scoop equal portions of *Filling* into center of one side of dough circle. Fold bare half of dough over filled half. Press edges together, letting any trapped air escape. Crimp edges of dough together with fork. Repeat with remaining dough.

8. Arrange pies on lined sheet pan and bake 15 - 20 minutes, or until dough is golden and cooked through.

9. Serve immediately.

*stevia, raw honey or agave nectar

NOTE: Heat large skillet over medium heat , add 1/4 inch coconut oil, and fry pies 2 minutes on each side for traditional *Fried Pies*.

Chocolate Fried Pie

Prep Time: 20 minutes*

Cook Time: 20 minutes

Servings: 4

INSTRUCTIONS

Crust

2 cups almond flour

2 eggs

3 tablespoons coconut oil

1 tablespoon sweetener*

1/4 teaspoon baking soda

1 tablespoon cocoa powder

1/2 teaspoon ground cinnamon

1/2 teaspoon sea salt

Filling

1 cup cashews*

1/2 cup dried dates*

1/4 cup coconut cream

3 tablespoons cocoa powder

1 egg

1 teaspoon vanilla

1 teaspoon ground cinnamon

1 teaspoon ground nutmeg

1/2 teaspoon ground black pepper

DIRECTIONS

1. *Soak cashew and dates for at least 4 hours in 2 cups water. Drain, then add all *Filling* ingredients to food processor or bullet blender and process until smooth. Set aside.

2. For *Crust*, sift almond flour into medium mixing bowl. Add baking soda, cocoa, cinnamon and salt.

3. Whisk eggs and sweetener in small mixing bowl, then add to flour and combine. Slowly add coconut oil until formable dough comes together.

4. Roll in plastic wrap or wrap tightly in parchment and refrigerate for 15 minutes.

5. Preheat oven to 400 degrees. Line sheet pan with parchment or baking mat.

6. Remove dough from refrigerator. Divide dough into 4 portions. Roll dough into balls and flatten on parchment covered cutting board with hands. Roll into circles about 1/8 inch thick with rolling pin.

7. Scoop equal portions of *Filling* into center of one side of dough circle. Fold bare half of dough over filled half. Press edges together, letting any trapped air escape. Crimp edges of dough together with fork. Repeat with remaining dough.

8. Arrange pies on lined sheet pan and bake 15 - 20 minutes, or until dough is golden and cooked through.

9. Serve immediately.

*stevia, raw honey or agave nectar

NOTE: Heat large skillet over medium heat , add 1/4 inch coconut oil, and fry pies 2 minutes on each side for traditional *Fried Pies*.

Chocolate Banana Bites

Prep Time: 10 minutes

Cook Time: 5 minutes

Servings: 1

INGREDIENTS

1 banana

2 - 4 oz organic bittersweet or semisweet chocolate

3 tablespoons chopped nuts (or flaked coconut)

DIRECTIONS

1. Heat chocolate over double boiler until melted, about 5 minutes.
2. Peel banana and cut in 1 inch slices.
3. Dip banana pieces into chocolate, or spread chocolate over tops of banana slices.
4. Sprinkle nuts or coconut over chocolate.
5. Place dipped, topped bananas in freezer for 5 minutes, or until chocolate is set.
6. Serve chilled.

NOTE: For *Frozen Chocolate Banana Bites*, leave dipped, topped banana pieces in freezer for 20 minutes, then serve.

Fruit 'N Nut Bars

Prep Time: 10 minutes

Cook Time: 10 minutes

Servings: 6

INGREDIENTS

1/4 cup dried cherries

1/2 cup dried apricots

1/4 cup dried cranberries

1/4 cup dried dates

1/3 cup warm water

1 cup cashews

1/2 teaspoon vanilla

1/2 teaspoon ground cinnamon

1/4 teaspoon ground ginger

1/4 teaspoon sea salt

INSTRUCTIONS

1. Soak dried fruit in warm water for 5 - 10 minutes. Drain and add to food processor or bullet blender with cashews, vanilla, cinnamon, ginger and salt.
2. Process until mixture forms a sticky mass, about 1 minute.
3. Transfer to loaf pan lined with parchment. Fold parchment over mixture and press firmly into bottom of pan with spatula or hand.
4. Refrigerate for 10 minutes. Remove and cut into 6 bars.
5. Serve chilled or room temperature.

Hoppin' Hot Chocolate

Prep Time: 5 minutes

Cook Time: 15 minutes

Servings: 4

INGREDIENTS

2 cups unsweetened nutmilk (not full-fat coconut milk)

13 oz (1 can) full-fat coconut milk

1/4 cup raw honey or agave nectar

4 oz bittersweet or baking chocolate

2 tablespoons cocoa powder

2 tablespoons instant espresso (or instant coffee)

1 tablespoon ground cinnamon

1 teaspoon vanilla

1 teaspoon ground black pepper

1/2 teaspoon ground cayenne pepper

INSTRUCTIONS

1. Add nutmilk, coconut milk and vanilla to medium pot. Heat over medium-high heat and bring to a boil. Reduce heat and simmer for 10 minutes.

2. Whisk in chocolate, sweetener, cocoa powder, espresso, cinnamon, pepper and cayenne. Whisk occasionally for 5 minutes, until chocolate is melted and mixture becomes thick and creamy.

3. Pour into mugs and serve warm.

Piña Colada Smoothie

Prep Time: 5 minutes

Cook Time: 5 minutes

Servings: 2

INSTRUCTIONS

1 large banana

1 cup pineapple chunks (fresh, frozen or canned)

2 tablespoons flaked coconut

1 cup coconut milk

1 cup ice (crushed preferably)

DIRECTIONS

1. Add banana, pineapple, coconut, coconut milk and ice to highs-speed blender. Process until smooth.
2. Pour into chilled glasses and serve immediately.

Spicy Chicken Bites

Prep Time: 5 minutes

Cook Time: 10 minutes

Servings: 4

INGREDIENTS

8 oz boneless skinless chicken

1/2 cup almond meal

1 teaspoon flax meal

1 teaspoon paprika

1/2 teaspoon cayenne pepper

1/2 teaspoon red pepper flakes

1/2 teaspoon ground black pepper

1/2 teaspoon sea salt

1 egg

1 jalapeño pepper

2 garlic cloves

2 oz organic spicy brown mustard

Coconut oil (for cooking)

INSTRUCTIONS

1. Heat a medium skillet over medium high heat. Lightly coat pan with coconut oil.
2. Slice chicken into 1x1 inch strips. Arrange slices between 2 sheets of parchment and pound with kitchen mallet or rolling pin to

flatten slightly. Place flattened pieces between two paper towels to absorb excess moisture.

3. In a shallow dish, blend almond meal, flax meal, dry spices and salt.

4. Add egg , jalapeño and peeled garlic to food processor or bullet blender. Process until fairly smooth. Pour into shallow dish.

5. Dip chicken pieces into jalapeño egg, then dredge in seasoned almond meal.

6. Carefully place coated chicken pieces into hot oil and fry about 2 minutes, until golden brown and cooked through. Turn with tongs half way through.

7. Drain cooked chicken on paper towel, then transfer to serving dish.

8. Serve hot with spicy mustard.

Highland Scotch Egg

Prep Time: 10 minutes

Cook Time: 25 minutes

Servings: 6

INGREDIENTS

6 eggs

12 oz ground sausage (pork, chicken, etc.)

1 tablespoon dried parsley

2 teaspoons lemon zest

1/4 teaspoon ground nutmeg

1/4 teaspoon dried sage

Pinch sea salt

Pinch ground black pepper

1 egg

1/2 cup almond meal

Coconut oil (for cooking)

Mustard Sauce

1 egg yolk

1/4 cup coconut oil

1/4 cup organic mustard

2 tablespoons sweetener*

INSTRUCTIONS

1. Bring medium pot of lightly salted water to boil.

2. Carefully place eggs in pot with tongs. Boil eggs for about 10 minutes.

3. For *Mustard Sauce*, add yolk, coconut oil, mustard and sweetener to food processor and bullet blender. Process until emulsified, about 2 minutes. Transfer to serving dish and refrigerate about 15 minutes.

4. Heat small pot over medium heat. Add enough coconut oil to cover width of whole egg, about 2 1/2 inches.

5. Drain eggs and cool under cold running water. Once cool, peel off shells and set aside.

6. Add sausage to medium bowl with parsley, lemon zest, nutmeg, sage, salt and pepper. Mix to combine.

7. Wet hands and cover each whole, peeled egg with a layer of seasoned sausage. Work sausage around eggs and pat into even layer.

8. Pour almond meal into shallow dish. Whisk egg in small bowl. Roll sausage covered eggs in beaten egg, then dredge in almond meal.

9. Carefully place 2 eggs into hot oil and fry for 4 to 5 minutes, until browned and heated through. Turn half way through cooking with tongs.

10. Remove eggs with tongs or slotted spoon and place on paper towel to drain. Repeat with remaining eggs.

11. Serve hot with *Mustard Sauce*.

stevia, raw honey or agave nectar

NOTE: For *Baked Scotch Eggs*, preheat oven to 400 degrees F and bake coated eggs on wire rack over sheet pan for about 15 minutes, until sausage is fully cooked.

Jalapeño Bacon Bites

Prep Time: 15 minutes

Cook Time: 20 minutes

Servings: 4

INGREDIENTS

6 medium to large jalapeño peppers

6 strips nitrate-free bacon

12 - 24 wooden toothpicks

Nut Cream Cheese

1/2 cup skinless almonds

1/2 cup cashews

2 tablespoons coconut oil

1 tablespoon lemon juice

1 tablespoon apple cider vinegar

1 garlic clove

1/4 teaspoon ground white pepper (or black pepper)

1/2 teaspoon sea salt

INSTRUCTIONS

1. Soak toothpicks in water for about 5 minutes.
2. Peel garlic, and add all *Nut Cream Cheese* ingredients to food processor or bullet blender. Process until smooth. If necessary, let mixture sit for a few minutes, then continue to process to reach desired consistency.

3. Preheat oven to 375 degrees F. Place oven-safe wire rack over sheet pan.

4. Slice jalapeños in half lengthwise. Remove stems, seeds and veins. Cut bacon strips in half.

5. Fill jalapeño wells with *Nut Cream Cheese*, then wrap in half slice of bacon. Use 1 or 2 toothpicks per jalapeño to secure bacon.

6. Place bacon wrapped pepper on wire rack filling side up and place in oven. Bake for about 15 - 20 minutes, or until bacon is crisp. Remove and let cool about 2 minutes.

7. Serve warm or room temperature.

Fried Green Tomatoes

Prep Time: 5 minutes

Cook Time: 15 minutes

Servings: 4

INGREDIENTS

2 large green tomatoes

Pinch sea salt

Pinch ground black pepper

Coconut oil (for cooking)

Coating

1 cup almond flour

1 tablespoon tapioca flour

1 tablespoon ground chia seed (or flax meal)

1 egg

1/2 cup nut milk

1/4 cup almond meal

1/4 cup almonds

1/4 teaspoon ground black pepper

1/2 teaspoon sea salt

INSTRUCTIONS

1. Heat medium pan over medium heat. Add 1/2 inch worth of coconut oil.

2. Slice tomatoes into 1/2 inch thick slices. Discard ends.

3. Grind 1/4 cup almonds into course meal in food processor or bullet blender. Do not process into almond butter. Add to 1/4 cup almond meal, 1/4 teaspoon black pepper and 1/2 teaspoon salt in shallow dish.

4. In separate dish, combine almond flour, tapioca flour, and chia or flax meal.

5. Whisk eggs and milk together in small mixing bowl.

6. Dip tomato slices into flour mixture to coat. Then into the egg and milk mixture. Then dredge into almond meal mixture.

7. Carefully place 4 or 5 well coated tomatoes at a time into hot oil. Fry tomatoes for 2 -3 minutes on each side, until golden. Drain on paper towel and repeat with remaining tomatoes.

8. Serve hot.

Bacon Mofongo

Prep Time: 15 minutes

Cook Time: 15 minutes

Servings: 2

INGREDIENTS

1 green plantain

2 slices nitrate-free bacon

3 garlic cloves

1/4 teaspoon ground black pepper

Bacon drippings

Coconut oil (for cooking)

INSTRUCTIONS

1. Bring medium pot of lightly salted water to boil.
2. Cut plantains into 1 inch slices. Remove peel and add to boiling water. Boil plantains for about 10 minutes, until soft.
3. Heat small pot over medium heat. Dice bacon and add to pot. Sauté and render out fat for about 5 minutes, until bacon is crisp. Pour bacon and drippings into medium bowl to cool slightly.
4. Add 1 inch worth of coconut oil to hot pot.
5. Add slightly cooled bacon and drippings to food processor or bullet blender with peeled garlic. Process until well blended. Add back to medium bowl. Drain plantains and add to bowl with black pepper.

6. Mash plantains and seasonings in bowl with fork or potato masher. Roll mixture into 6 small balls.

7. Carefully add plantain balls to hot oil and fry for about 2 minutes. Turn with tongs half way through cooking. Remove and drain on paper towel.

8. Serve hot.

NOTE: For *Baked Mofongo*, preheat oven to 400 degrees F and bake plantain balls on oiled or parchment covered sheet pan for about 10 minutes, until golden brown.

Simple Guacamole

Prep Time: 5 minutes

Cook Time: 5 minutes

Servings: 4

INGREDIENTS

2 avocados

1 shallot

1 small tomato

1 bunch cilantro

Half lime

2 teaspoons paprika

1/2 teaspoon ground cumin

1/2 teaspoon ground black pepper

1/2 teaspoon sea salt

INSTRUCTIONS

1. Peel and finely dice shallot. Dice tomato and cilantro. Add to small mixing bowl.
2. Slice avocados in half, pit, and scoop flesh into bowl. Add 1 teaspoon paprika, 1/2 teaspoon cumin, 1/2 teaspoon black pepper and 1/2 teaspoon salt.
3. Mash avocado and mix ingredients well with fork. Transfer to serving dish and squeeze on juice of half a lime. Sprinkle with remaining teaspoon of paprika.
4. Serve immediately. Or refrigerate 30 minutes, and serve chilled.

Coconut Shrimp

Prep Time: 10 minutes

Cook Time: 15 minutes

Servings: 4

INGREDIENTS

3 egg whites

1 lb large shrimp

1 cup flaked coconut

1/2 teaspoon garlic powder

1/2 teaspoon ground white pepper (or ground black pepper)

1 teaspoon sea salt

Coconut oil (for cooking)

Mango Salsa

1 ripe mango

1/2 small white onion

1 small jalapeño

Juice of half lime

INSTRUCTIONS

1. Preheat oven to 425 degrees F. Line sheet pan with parchment paper. Or place oven-safe wire rack over sheet pan.
2. Add coconut to shallow dish.
3. Beat egg whites with salt, pepper and garlic powder in a large mixing bowl with hand mixer or whisk until light and fluffy.

4. Peel and devein shrimp. Leave tails on. Add shrimp to egg whites to coat.

5. Let excess egg white drain from shrimp, then add to coconut flakes. Toss to coat. Return shrimp to egg whites, then coconut flakes again. Press shrimp into coconut and coat well.

6. Place the shrimp on prepared sheet pan. Brush lightly with liquid coconut oil.

7. Place in oven and bake for 5 - 7 minutes. Then turn shrimp over, brush with coconut oil, and bake another 5 - 7 minutes, until coconut is golden brown and shrimp are bright pink.

8. For *Mango Salsa*, slice mango around pit. Peel and dice flesh. Peel and dice onion. Mince jalapeño, discarding seeds and stem. Add to small serving dish juice of half a lime. Mix to combine.

9. Remove shrimp from oven and allow to cool for a few minutes.

10. Serve warm with *Mango Salsa*.

Green Deviled Eggs 'N Ham

Prep Time: 5 minutes

Cook Time: 10 minutes

Servings: 4

INGREDIENTS

8 eggs

1 avocado

1/2 teaspoon ground black pepper

1/2 teaspoon salt

2 oz natural ham

2 tablespoons fresh dill

INSTRUCTIONS

1. Bring medium pot of lightly salted water to boil. Gently add eggs to hot water with tongs and cook about 8 - 10 minutes.
2. Drain eggs in colander and cool in cold water.
3. Crack shells and peel eggs. Cut eggs in half lengthwise and scoop out yolks into small bowl. Arrange whites on platter with center hollows facing up.
4. Mash avocado, salt and pepper with egg yolks until smooth. Dice ham and dill, separately.
5. Scoop avocado blend into each egg white hollow and sprinkle with ham, then dill.
6. Refrigerate about 20 minutes. Serve chilled.

Zucchini Rollatini

Prep Time: 15 minutes*

Cook Time: 25 minutes

Servings: 4

INGREDIENTS

Zucchini Pasta

1 large zucchini

Pinch sea salt

Pinch ground black pepper

Cashew Ricotta

1 cup cashews

1 1/2 cups water

2 teaspoons fresh basil

1 teaspoon ground white pepper (or black pepper)

1/2 teaspoon garlic powder

1/2 teaspoon sea salt

Pasta Sauce

6 oz (1 can) organic tomato paste

1/4 cup water

1 garlic clove

1 tablespoon oregano

2 teaspoons paprika

1 teaspoon ground black pepper

1/2 teaspoon sea salt

INSTRUCTIONS

1. *For *Cashew Ricotta*, soak cashews for at least 4 hours in 1 1/2 cups water. Drain and rinse. Process with basil, white pepper, garlic powder and salt in food processor or bullet blender until smooth. Add water 1 tablespoon at a time as necessary. Set aside.
2. Preheat oven to 350 degrees F. Bring medium pot of lightly salted water to boil. Line square baking pan with parchment, or lightly coat with coconut oil.
3. For *Pasta Sauce*, process all sauce ingredients in food processor or bullet blender, then pour into small pot. Heat over medium heat and stir until warm. Remove from heat and set aside.
4. Slice zucchini into thin wide strips with sharp knife or mandolin. Blanch zucchini sheets in boiling water for about 30 seconds, just to make pliable. Remove and lay on paper towel or parchment. Sprinkle with pinch of salt and pepper.
5. Spread *Pasta Sauce* on zucchini. Place dollop of *Cashew Ricotta* toward one end of zucchini sheet. Roll up zucchini around ricotta until fully rolled.
6. Place rolled zucchini in lined baking sheet and bake for about 15 minutes, until heated through.
7. Remove from oven and serve hot.

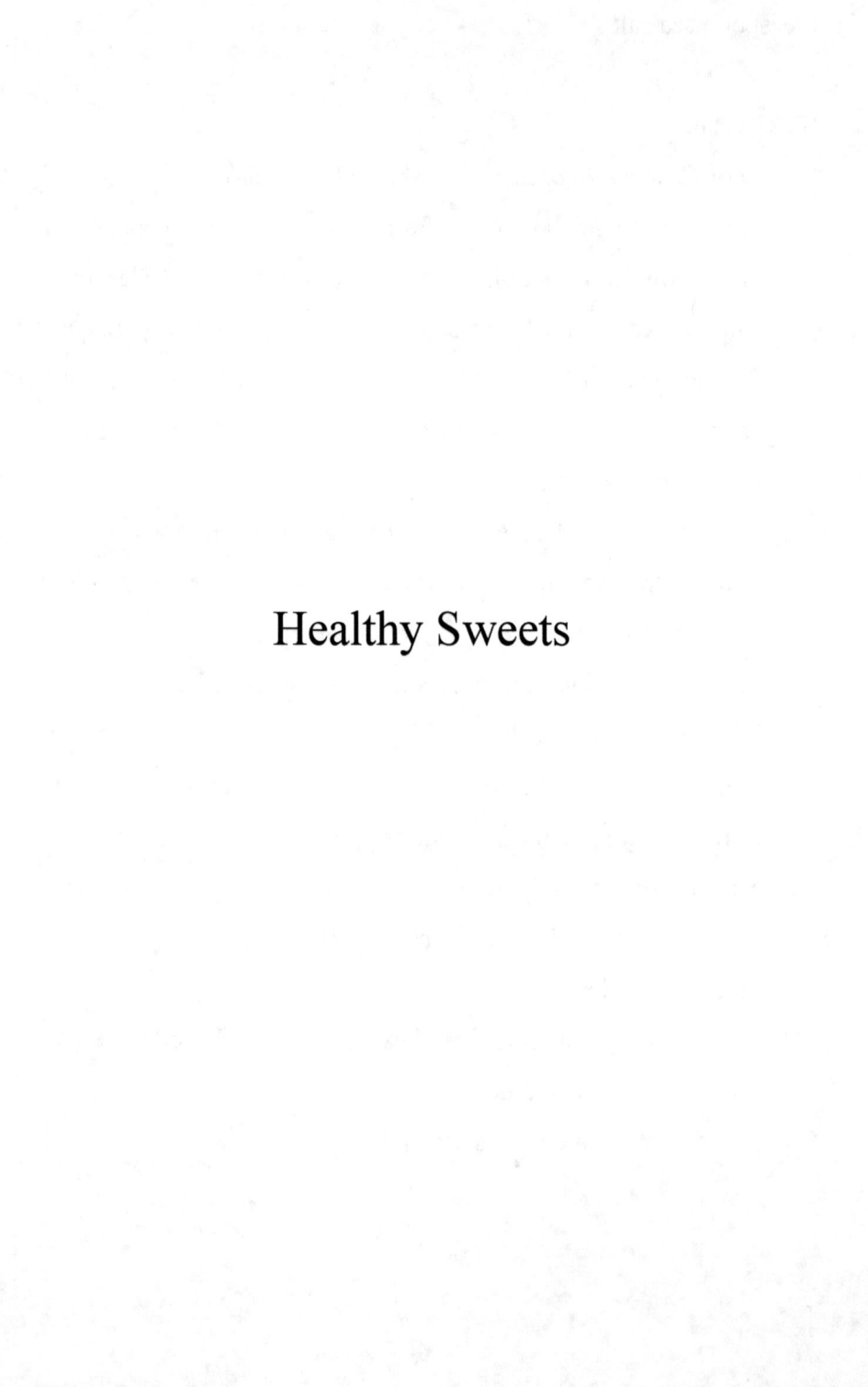

Healthy Sweets

Frozen Chocolate Cherry Custard

Prep Time: 15* minutes

Cook Time: 20 minutes

Servings: 4

INGREDIENTS

13 oz (1 can) full-fat coconut milk

3 oz water

5 egg yolks

1/4 cup sweetener*

1/2 cup pitted cherries

3 tablespoons cocoa powder

2 teaspoons vanilla

INSTRUCTIONS

1. *Freeze ice cream maker canister overnight before to make sure it is cold enough.
2. Heat coconut milk and water in medium pan over medium heat.
3. Slice cherries in half and set aside.
4. While milk is warmed, but not hot, whisk in egg yolks, sweetener and vanilla. Blend well.
5. Sift in cocoa powder and continue whisking until thickened, about 5 minutes.
6. Turn on ice cream maker first, then carefully pour in custard as ice cream maker paddle rotates.
7. Add halved cherries as ice cream maker runs.

8. Freeze mixture about 15 - 20 minutes. Then transfer frozen custard to serving dishes.
9. Serve immediately.

stevia, raw honey, agave nectar or maple syrup

Sugar Cookies

Prep Time: 10 minutes

Cook Time: 15 minutes

Servings: 12

INGREDIENTS

1 1/2 cups almond flour

1 cup coconut flour

1/2 cup sweetener*

5 dried pitted dates

1 egg

2 teaspoons coconut oil

1 teaspoon vanilla

1/2 teaspoon baking soda

Pinch sea salt

Water

INSTRUCTIONS

1. Preheat oven to 350 degrees F. Line sheet pan with parchment paper. Bring small pot of water to boil. Add dates and boil for about 5 - 8 minutes, until softened.

2. Add dates to food processor or bullet blender and process until smooth. Add leftover water if necessary.

3. Add sweetener, egg, oil and vanilla to dates and process until smooth.

4. Add date mixture to medium bowl. Sift in almond flour, coconut flour baking soda and salt. Beat with hand mixer until combined and smooth, about 5 minutes.

5. Roll dough into a log about 3 inches in diameter. Slice into 1/4 inch thick disks.

6. Place disks on sheet pan and bake for about 8 - 10 minutes.

7. Remove form oven and cool for a few minutes.

8. Serve warm or room temperature.

*stevia, raw honey or agave nectar

Carrot Cake Cookies
Prep Time: 10 minutes

Cook Time: 20 minutes

Servings: 12

INGREDIENTS

2 cups almond meal

4 large carrots (2 cups shredded)

3 eggs

1/4 cup coconut oil

1/3 cup unsweetened applesauce

1/2 cup coconut flakes

1/4 cup pitted dates

2 teaspoons vanilla

2 teaspoons ground cinnamon

1 teaspoon ground nutmeg

1 teaspoon ground ginger

INSTRUCTIONS

1. Preheat your oven to 350 Degrees F. Line sheet pan with parchment sheet or coat lightly with coconut oil.
2. Grate carrots, or process in food processor or bullet blender until finely chopped. Add to medium bowl.
3. Add eggs, oil, applesauce and dates to food processor or bullet blender. Process until thick, slightly chunky mixture forms. Pour into carrots.

4. Sift in almond meal. Then add spices and vanilla. Mix well with a wooden spoon. Stir in coconut.

5. Form 12 round balls and evenly space on sheet pan. Flatten balls with hand.

6. Bake about 20 minutes, or until firm and golden brown.

7. Remove from oven and allow to cool about 5 minutes.

8. Serve warm or room temperature.

raw honey, agave nectar or maple syrup

Chocolate Mousse

Prep Time: 5 minutes

Cook Time: 5 minutes

Servings: 2

INGREDIENTS

1 3/4 cups (about 2 cans) full-fat coconut milk

1 avocado

1/3 cup sweetener*

2 tablespoons cocoa powder

1 teaspoon vanilla

Handful cacao nibs or chapped nuts (optional)

INSTRUCTIONS

1. Process coconut milk, sweetener, cacao powder and vanilla in food processor or bullet blender until well combined.
2. Slice avocado in half and pit. Scoop flesh into mixture. Process until thick and creamy.
3. Stir in *optional* cacao nibs, nuts, etc.
4. Pour into ramekins or dessert cups and serve immediately. Or refrigerate for 1 hour to thicken.
5. Serve room temperature or chilled.

raw honey, agave nectar or maple syrup

Banana Bread Pudding

Prep Time: 10 minutes

Cook Time: 30 minutes

Servings: 12

INGREDIENTS

Banana Bread

1 cup of almond flour

2 eggs

2 overripe bananas

1/4 cup sweetener*

2 tablespoons coconut oil

1 tablespoon baking powder

1 tablespoon cinnamon

1 teaspoon nutmeg

1 teaspoon vanilla

1/2 teaspoon of sea salt

Banana Custard

13 oz (1 can) full-fat coconut milk

6 egg yolks

1 overripe banana

1/4 cup sweetener*

1/4 cup raisins

1/2 cup dried pitted dates

2 tablespoons tapioca starch/flour

2 teaspoons vanilla

1 teaspoon cinnamon

Pinch sea salt

INSTRUCTIONS

1. Preheat oven to 350 degrees F. Line muffin pan with paper liners or coat with coconut oil.
2. In medium mixing bowl, beat 2 eggs, 2 bananas, 2 tablespoons oil and 1/4 cup sweetener with hand mixer or whisk.
3. In separate mixing bowl, add 1 cup almond flour, 1 tablespoon baking powder,1 tablespoon cinnamon, 1 teaspoon nutmeg, 1 teaspoon vanilla and 1/2 teaspoon salt.
4. Pour banana mixture into flour mixture and mix well.
5. Pour batter into muffin pan and bake for about 15 minutes, or until golden brown, risen and firm.
6. While muffins cook, add coconut milk, egg yolks, banana, sweetener, vanilla, cinnamon and salt to medium bowl and blend briefly with hand mixer or whisk.
7. Pour into medium pot and heat over medium heat. Chop dates and add to pot with raisins.
8. Stir in tapioca flour. Stir as *Banana Custard* thickens, about 5 minutes. Remove from heat.
9. Remove muffins from oven and turn out onto cutting board.
10. Increase oven to 375 degrees F. Lightly coat square or rectangular baking dish with coconut oil.

11. Carefully remove paper liners and roughly chop muffins. Add muffin chunks to baking dish. Pour banana custard over chopped muffins.
12. Place dish in oven and bake for 15 minutes.
13. Remove and allow to cool for 15 minutes before serving.
14. Serve warm or room temperature.

stevia, raw honey or agave nectar

Mixed Berry Trifle

Prep Time: 10 minutes

Cook Time: 25 minutes

Servings: 12

INGREDIENTS

Cake

1 cup almond flour

1 cup coconut flour

3/4 cup coconut milk

4 eggs

1/2 cup sweetener*

1/2 cup coconut oil

2 tablespoons vanilla

2 teaspoons baking soda

Filling

1 cup coconut cream

2 tablespoons sweetener*

1 cup strawberries

1/2 cup blueberries

1/2 cup raspberries

1/2 cup blackberries

Juice of orange half

Juice of lemon half

Zest of orange half

Zest of lemon half

1/4 cup pistachios

INSTRUCTIONS

1. Preheat oven to 350 degrees F. Line muffin pan with paper liner or coat with coconut oil.
2. In large mixing bowl, beat eggs and coconut milk until light and airy. Beat in sweetener, oil and vanilla.
3. Sift in almond flour, coconut flour and baking soda. Mix until well combined.
4. Use ice cream scoop or spoon to scoop batter into muffin pan. Fill each cup 1/2 - 2/3 full with batter.
5. Bake in for about 15 minutes, until firm but springy in the center.
6. Remove cupcakes from oven and turn out onto wire rack or plate. Allow to cool for about 10 minutes and remove paper liners.
7. Dice strawberries and add to medium bowl with blueberries, raspberries, blackberries, lemon and orange zests and juices. Toss to combine.
8. In small bowl, mixi coconut cream with 2 tablespoon sweetener.
9. Slice cupcake in half to create top and bottom. Dollop coconut cream onto bottom half, then top with a spoonful of fruit. Drain juice from spoon before adding to cake.
10. Place cupcake top on top of fruit. Press down slightly. Add another dollop of coconut cream and another spoonful of fruit. Repeat with remaining cupcakes.
11. Serve room temperature. Or chill for 30 minutes and serve.

NOTE: Bake cake in 3 round cake pans for 20 minutes, then layer with cream and berries and stack for **Mixed Berry Trifle Cake**.

*stevia, raw honey or agave nectar

Tapioca Blueberry Crepes

Prep Time: 5 minutes

Cook Time: 15 minutes

Servings: 2

INGREDIENTS

Crêpes:

1 cup tapioca flour/starch

1 cup coconut milk

1 egg

Pinch sea salt

Coconut oil (for cooking)

Filling:

1 pint blueberries

2 tablespoons sweetener*

1 teaspoon vanilla

Pinch ground black pepper

Pinch sea salt

1 tablespoon water

Topping:

1/2 cup coconut crème

2 tablespoons agave nectar

1/2 teaspoon vanilla

Coconut milk (for thinning)

INSTRUCTIONS

1. Heat large non-stick pan over medium heat. Add small dollop of coconut oil and carefully spread with wadded paper towel to coat evenly . Preserve paper towel.
2. Heat medium pan over medium heat. Add all **Filling** ingredients except water. Stir occasionally with wooden spoon. Add extra tablespoon of water if blueberries do not break down enough. Remove from heat when sufficiently warmed and saucy.
3. Combine all **Crêpe** ingredients in a medium bowl. Blend thoroughly.
4. When large non-stick pan is hot, use ladle or dry measure cup to pour in 1/3 cup of crêpe batter while tilting pan in all directions to evenly spread batter.
5. Cook crêpe about 2 minutes, then carefully flip and cook another 1 - 2 minutes.
6. When both sides are lightly browned, remove crêpe to plate and oil pan with wadded paper towel. Repeat process of cooking crêpe and oiling pan with remaining batter.
7. Blend all **Topping** ingredients. Thin with small amount of coconut milk to create drizzling consistency if necessary.
8. Fill crêpes with blueberry compote down center and fold over each side. Plate fold-side down and drizzle on coconut crème **Topping**. Serve warm.

*stevia, raw honey, or agave nectar

Raw Cocoa Chutney

Prep Time: 5 minutes*

Servings: 4

INGREDIENTS

10 oz (1 package) dried pitted dates

2 cups water

2 - 4 tablespoons raw cacao powder

1/2 teaspoon ground cinnamon

1/2 teaspoon black pepper

INSTRUCTIONS

1. *Soak dates in water over night. Drain and reserve 1/2 cup liquid.

2. Add soaked dates to medium mixing bowl. Add cacao powder and mash with large fork or potato masher for about 5 minutes, until chunky mixture forms.

3. Add soaking liquid or more cacao powder to reach desired consistency, texture and taste.

4. Add spices and mix until combined.

5. Transfer to serving dish and serve with fruits, veggies or raw breads.

Red Ants On A Log

Prep Time: 5 minutes

Servings: 2

INGREDIENTS

3 celery stalks

2 tablespoons dried cranberries

Cashew Butter

1 cup cashews

1 dried pitted date

1 teaspoon raw virgin coconut oil

1/2 teaspoon ground cinnamon

1/4 teaspoon sea salt

INSTRUCTIONS

1. Add cashews, date, cinnamon, salt and coconut oil to food processor or bullet blender. Process until smooth. Let mixture rest between periods of processing to reach desired consistency, if necessary.

2. Cut celery stalks into thirds and fill wells with *Cashew Butter*. Place cranberries on cashew butter.

3. Serve room temperature. Or refrigerate 10 minutes and serve chilled.

Raw Fudge

Prep Time: 10* minutes

Servings: 6

INGREDIENTS

1/4 cup raw cacao powder

3/4 cup raw almonds

1/2 cup raw hazelnuts (or cashews)

2 tablespoons raw virgin coconut oil

1/4 cup raw honey

1/4 cup hazelnuts (or walnuts)

INSTRUCTIONS

1. Line square baking dish with parchment paper.
2. Process almonds, 1/2 cup hazelnuts and coconut oil in food processor or bullet blender. Blend until fairly smooth and creamy.
3. Add nut butter, cocoa powder and honey to medium mixing bowl and mix well.
4. Chop remaining nuts.
5. *Spread mixture into parchment lined baking dish and top with chopped nuts. Refrigerate for 2 - 3 hours, until completely set.
6. Slice and serve chilled or room temperature.

Raw Banana Cream Pie

Prep Time: 10 minutes*

Servings: 8

INGREDIENTS

Crust

1 cup raw cashews

1 cup unsweetened flaked or shredded coconut

1/2 cup dried pitted dates

1/4 teaspoon vanilla

1/4 teaspoon sea salt

Filling

2 ripe bananas

3/4 cup raw cashews

1/3 cup raw virgin coconut oil

1/4 cup raw honey

Juice of 2 lemons

1 teaspoon vanilla

Pinch teaspoon sea salt

INSTRUCTIONS

1. Place all *Crust* ingredients in food processor or high-speed blender. Process until well broken down and mixture sticks together.

2. Divide crust mixture among 4 mini pie pans. Press the crust firmly into dish your hands. Place crusts in freezer.

3. Peel bananas and add to clean food processor or blender. Juice lemons and add to processor with cashews, coconut oil, honey, vanilla and salt. Process until creamy and smooth.

4. Pour banana cream filling onto chilled crusts. Smooth tops with spatula or back of a spoon.

5. Cover pies with parchment and place in freezer for at least 30 minutes before serving.

6. Serve chilled.

7. Store leftovers in freezer.

NOTE: Press crust into single large pie pan, fill with filling and freeze for at least 3 hours for large **Raw Banana Cream Pie**.

Date Butter and Apples

Prep Time: 5 minutes*

Servings: 2

INGREDIENTS

1 cup dried pitted dates

2 cups water

1 teaspoon ground cinnamon

1/4 teaspoon ground ginger

1/4 teaspoon ground white pepper (or ground black pepper)

2 tart apples

INSTRUCTIONS

1. *Soak dates overnight in water. Drain and reserve soaking liquid.
2. Add soaked dates and spices to food processor or high-speed blender with 1/4 cup reserved liquid. Process on high until thick paste forms. Add more reserved liquid to thin mixture if necessary.
3. Core and slice apples
4. Transfer date butter to serving dish and serve with apple slices.

Almond Butter Balls

Prep Time: 20 minutes

Servings: 12

INGREDIENTS

1 cup raw almonds

2 - 4 tablespoon raw honey

1 tablespoon raw virgin coconut oil (or almond oil)

1 tablespoon raw cacao powder (plus extra)

1 tablespoon ground chia seed (or flax meal)

1 teaspoon cinnamon

1/2 teaspoon sea salt

INSTRUCTIONS

1. Add whole chia seeds or flax to bullet blender or spice grinder and grind to fine powder.

2. Add chia or flax meal to food processor or bullet blender with almonds, coconut oil, honey, cocoa powder, cinnamon and salt.

3. Process into smooth, thick paste. Let mixture rest between periods of processing to reach desired consistency, if necessary.

4. Spread mixture in parchment lined dish. Place in refrigerator or freezer for 10 minutes.

5. Remove mixture and scoop and roll into balls. Roll in extra cacao powder and serve.

Red Berry Smoothie

Prep Time: 5 minutes

Servings: 1

INGREDIENTS

1 cup strawberries

1/2 cup red raspberries

1/4 cup pitted cherries

1/4 cup cherry tomatoes

1/2 - 1 cup water (or fresh nut milk)

Juice of 1 beet (optional)

INSTRUCTIONS

1. Remove leaves from strawberries and chop. Add to full sized blender with raspberries, cherries, tomatoes and beet juice (optional).
2. Add 1/2 cup water and pulse on low for 30 seconds to break down. Add more water if necessary. Then process on high for 30 seconds to 1 minute, until smooth.
3. Pour into serving glasses and serve immediately.
4. Or chill in refrigerator for 20 minutes, blend for a few seconds to incorporate separated liquid, then pour into serving glasses and serve chilled.

Strawberry Banana Shake

Prep Time: 5 minutes*

Cook Time: 0 minutes

Servings: 1

INGREDIENTS

1 banana

1 cup strawberries

1/2 - 1 cup water

Meat of 1/2 fresh coconut (or 1/2 cup unsweetened flaked or shredded coconut)

INSTRUCTIONS

1. *Soak flaked coconut in water for at least 4 hours.
2. Add fresh or soaked flaked coconut and water to high-speed blender. Process on high until smooth, about 1 minute.
3. Strain coconut mixture through nut milk bag or a few layers of cheese cloth. Squeeze out all excess liquid. Reserve coconut milk. Dry excess coconut, process until finely ground, and use as coconut flour.
4. Remove leaves from strawberries and chop. Peel banana.
5. Add coconut milk to blender with fruit and process on high until smooth.
6. Pour into serving glass and serve immediately.

7. Or chill in refrigerator for 20 minutes, blend for a few seconds to incorporate separated liquid, then pour into serving glass and serve chilled.

Raw Coconut Chia pudding

Prep Time: 5 minutes*

Servings: 4

INGREDIENTS

2 cups water

Meat of 1 fresh coconut (or 1 cup unsweetened flaked or shredded coconut)

1/4 - 1/2 cup raw honey (or dried pitted dates)

1/4 cup whole chia seeds

1/4 cup unsweetened flaked or shredded coconut

1 teaspoon vanilla

INSTRUCTIONS

1. *Soak flaked coconut and dates (optional) in water for at least 4 hours.

2. Add fresh or soaked flaked coconut, water and dates (optional) to high-speed blender. Process on high until smooth, about 1 minute.

3. Strain coconut mixture through nut milk bag or a few layers of cheese cloth. Squeeze out all excess liquid. Reserve coconut milk. Dry excess coconut, process until finely ground, and use as coconut flour.

4. Add coconut milk, raw honey (if preferred), chia, shredded coconut and vanilla to medium mixing bowl. Whisk until well combined.

5. Pour into serving dishes and serve immediately.

6. Or chill in refrigerator for 20 minutes and serve chilled.

Milano Cookie Sandwiches

Prep Time: 30 minutes

Cook Time: 15 minutes

Servings: 12

INGREDIENTS

Lady Fingers

1/3 cup coconut flour

3 tablespoons arrowroot powder

4 eggs

1/4 cup sweetener*

1/2 teaspoon baking powder

1/2 teaspoon vanilla

Chocolate Filling

4 oz organic dark chocolate

2 oz full-fat coconut milk

INSTRUCTIONS

1. Preheat oven to 400 degrees F. Line two sheet pans with parchment paper. Fit pastry bag with 1/2 inch round tip, or cut 1/4 inch corner off sturdy kitchen storage bag (like Ziploc®).
2. For *Lady Fingers*, beat egg yolks, sweetener and vanilla until thick and pale.
3. In separate bowl, beat egg whites to stiff peaks with hand mixer or whisk, about 8 minutes. Fold half of egg whites into egg yolk

mixture. Then sift in coconut flour, arrowroot powder and baking powder. Fold in remaining egg whites.

4. Scoop batter into pastry or storage bag. Place in tall wide contain and fold open end of bag over edge of container for easier prep.

5. Pipe 4 inch cookies onto prepared sheet pans about 2 inches apart.

6. Place in oven and bake for 8 minutes, until set and just golden.

7. Remove cookies from oven and transfer full parchment sheet onto wire rack to cool completely. Do not try to remove warm cookies from parchment.

8. Heat 1 inch water in bottom of double boiler, or in bottom pan with metal or class bowl on top.

9. For Chocolate Filling, melt chocolate and coconut milk over double boiler until smooth.

10. Remove cooled *Lady Fingers* from parchment. Dip bottom of cookie in melted chocolate and press against bottom of second cookie to make sandwich. Repeat with remaining cookies.

11. Serve warm. Let chocolate set for 10 minutes, in refrigerator if preferred, and serve chilled or room temperature.

*stevia, raw honey or agave nectar

Berry Tart

Prep Time: 20 minutes

Cook Time: 25 minutes

Servings: 4

INGREDIENTS

Tart Shell

2 cups almond flour

1 egg

2 tablespoons coconut oil

1/2 teaspoon vanilla

1/2 teaspoon sea salt

Filling

1/2 cup coconut cream (settled from1 can full-fat coconut milk)

1/4 - 1/2 cup sweetener*

1/2 teaspoon vanilla

1/4 cup fresh blueberries

1/4 cup fresh sliced strawberries

1/4 cup fresh blackberries

1/4 cup fresh raspberries

INSTRUCTIONS

1. Preheat oven to 350 degrees F. Coat four 4-inch tart pans or pie plates with coconut oil.

2. For *Tart Shell*, add almond flour, salt and vanilla to food processor or high-speed blender and process about 30 seconds.

3. Add coconut oil and egg, and process until dough comes together.

4. Press dough into prepared pans and place in oven. Bake 8 - 10 minutes, or until golden brown. Remove pie shells from oven and set aside. Refrigerate to speed cooling.

5. For *Filling*, beat coconut cream, sweetener and vanilla with hand mixer or whisk in medium mixing bowl until thickened, about 2 minutes.

6. Pour cream mixture into *Tart Shells*. Top with fresh berries.

7. Serve immediately. Or refrigerate 20 minutes and serve chilled.

stevia, raw honey or agave nectar

NOTE: Bake crust in 9-inch tart pan for 12 - 15 minutes and fill for large **Berry Tart**.

Simple Strawberry Cake

Prep Time: 15 minutes

Cook Time: 30 minutes

Servings: 12

INGREDIENTS

2 cups almond flour

3 eggs

1 1/2 cups whole strawberries

1/4 cup sweetener*

1/4 cup coconut oil

2 teaspoons baking soda

1 teaspoon vanilla

1/2 teaspoon sea salt

INSTRUCTIONS

1. Preheat oven to 350 degrees F. Line 9 x 13 baking dish with parchment paper, or coat with coconut oil.

2. Add eggs to food processor or high-speed blender and process until light and thickened, about 1 minute. Remove stems from strawberries and roughly chop. Add to processor with sweetener, coconut oil and vanilla. Process until smooth.

3. Sift almond flour, baking soda and salt into medium mixing bowl. Pour in strawberry mixture and beat with hand mixer or whisk until well combined.

4. Pour batter into prepared baking pan and place in oven.

5. Bake 25 - 30 minutes, or until cake is golden brown on top and toothpick inserted into center comes out moist but clean.
6. Remove pan from oven and allow to cool 10 minutes.
7. Slice and serve warm. Or let cool completely and serve room temperature or warm.

NOTE: Line muffin pan with paper liners of light coat with coconut oil, fill 2/3 full with batter, and bake about 15 minutes for **Strawberry Cupcakes**.

*stevia, raw honey or agave nectar

Red Velvet Cupcakes

Prep Time: 10 minutes

Cook Time: 15 minutes

Servings: 12

INGREDIENTS

Red Velvet Cake

6 eggs

1 cup coconut flour

1/2 cup dried pitted dates

1/2 cup coconut oil

1/2 cup sweetener*

1/3 cup applesauce

1/4 cup cocoa powder

Juice of 1 beet

2 teaspoons vanilla

1 teaspoon baking soda

1 teaspoon sea salt

1 cup water

Coconut Cream Topping

1/2 cup coconut cream (settled from 1 can full-fat coconut milk)

1/4 - 1/2 cup sweetener*

1/2 teaspoon vanilla

1/3 cup walnuts (3 tablespoons finely chopped)

INSTRUCTIONS

1. Preheat oven to 350 degrees F. Line muffin pan with paper liners or lightly coat with coconut oil. Bring 1 cup water to boil in small pan.

2. Add dried dates to boiling water for about 5 minutes. Juice beet and set aside.

3. For *Red Velvet Cake*, sift flour, cocoa, baking soda and salt into small bowl.

4. In medium bowl, beat eggs until thick and frothy, about 5 minutes.

5. Add dates with just enough hot water to food processor or high-speed blender to process into thick paste.

6. Add date paste, sweetener, applesauce, coconut oil, beet juice and vanilla to eggs. Beat with hand mixer or whisk until combined.

7. Beat flour mixture into egg mixture until well combined.

8. Use ice cream scoop or spoon to pour batter into prepared muffin pan.

9. Place in oven and bake 15 - 20 minutes, until toothpick inserted into center comes out moist but clean.

10. For *Coconut Cream Topping*, beat coconut milk, sweetener and vanilla in medium mixing bowl with hand mixer or whisk until thick and fluffy. Refrigerate.

11. Finely chop walnuts. Set aside.

12. Remove muffin pan from oven and let cool at least 10 minutes. Place in refrigerator to speed cooling if desired.

13. Beat *Coconut Cream Topping* with hand mix or whisk again before frosting cakes.

14. Frost cooled cakes and serve room temperature.

raw honey, agave nectar or maple syrup

Primal Piña Colada Bars

Prep Time: 15 minutes

Cook Time: 30 minutes

Servings: 12

INGREDIENTS

Crust

1/2 cup raw cashews

2/3 cup coconut flour

2 eggs

2 tablespoons coconut oil

2 tablespoons sweetener*

1 tablespoon flaked or shredded coconut

1 teaspoon coconut milk

1/2 teaspoon baking soda

1/2 teaspoon vanilla

Filling

2 eggs

2 egg yolks

1 1/3 cups chopped pineapple (canned organic chunks in juice or fresh)

1/4 cup sweetener* (optional)

1/2 cup flaked or shredded coconut

2 tablespoons coconut flour

INSTRUCTIONS

1. Preheat oven to 350 degrees F. Lightly coat rectangular baking dish with coconut oil, or line with parchment.

2. For *Crust*, add cashews and coconut to food processor or high-speed blender and process until finely ground. Add remaining *Crust* ingredients to food processor and pulse until dough comes together.

3. Press dough into bottom of baking dish, and slightly up the sides. Dock crust with fork to prevent bubbling.

4. Place crust in oven and bake 8 - 10 minutes.

5. For *Filling*, add pineapple chunks to clean food processor or high-speed blender and process until fairly smooth.

6. Add processed pineapple to medium mixing bowl with eggs, egg yolks and sweetener (optional). Beat with hand mixer or whisk until well combined.

7. Sift in coconut flour and mix to combine. Let mixture sit for 5 minutes. Add flaked coconut and beat again to combine.

8. Pour *Filling* over par baked crust. Place in oven and bake 20 minutes, until center is set but still jiggles slightly.

9. Remove from oven and let cool for 20 minutes. Then place in refrigerate about 20 minutes, until fully set and chilled.

10. Slice and serve chilled or room temperature.

*stevia, raw honey or agave nectar

Sesame Logs

Prep Time: 10 minutes

Cook Time: 20 minutes

Servings: 12

INGREDIENTS

1 3/4 cups almond flour

1 egg

1 cup slightly melted cacao butter (or coconut oil)

1 cup dried pitted dates

1 cup sesame seeds

1/4 - 1/2 cup nut milk

2 teaspoons tahini (sesame butter)

1/4 teaspoon baking powder

1/4 teaspoon sea salt

INSTRUCTIONS

1. Preheat oven to 350 degrees F. Line sheet pan with parchment paper or baking mat.

2. Add cocoa butter or coconut oil, egg, tahini and dates to food processor or high-speed blender. Process for 1 minute, until thick and creamy.

3. In medium mixing bowl, sift together flour, baking powder and salt. Pour in date mixture and mix with hand mixer or whisk for about a minute, until light, thick dough forms.

4. Form dough into 1 inch circles. Then roll dough into logs. Add nut milk and sesame seeds to separate small dishes. Dip logs in nut milk, then roll in sesame seeds. Place on prepared sheet pan.

5. Place in oven and bake 15 - 20 minutes, or until bottom and sides are toasted.

6. Remove from oven and transfer to wire racks. Allow to cool completely.

7. Serve room temperature.

Chocolate Bacon Donut

Prep Time: 5 minutes

Cook Time: 20 minutes

Servings: 6

INGREDIENTS

Donuts

1 3/4 cups almond flour

1 tablespoon coconut flour

3 tablespoons cocoa powder

2 eggs

1/3 cup coconut oil

1/4 cup unsweetened applesauce

1/4 cup sweetener*

2 tablespoons nut milk (or water)

1 teaspoon baking soda

1 teaspoon vanilla

1/2 teaspoon sea salt

1/4 teaspoon ground black pepper (optional)

Topping

4 slices nitrate-free bacon

4 oz organic chocolate

2 tablespoons full-fat coconut milk

1 teaspoon cocoa powder

INSTRUCTIONS

1. Preheat oven to 350 degrees F. Lightly coat donut pan with coconut oil.
2. Add almond and coconut flours, cocoa, vanilla, baking soda, salt and pepper (optional) to food processor or high-speed blender. Process for 1 minute.
3. Add eggs, sweetener, coconut oil, applesauce, and nut milk. Process until airy batter forms, about 1 - 2 minutes.
4. Pour batter into donut pan until wells are 3/4 full.
5. Place in oven and bake for about 20 minutes, until dough is set and lightly browned.
6. For *Topping*, heat medium skillet over medium heat. Heat small pot over medium heat.
7. Chop bacon and add to hot skillet. Sauté until bacon is crisp and cooked through, about 5 minutes.
8. Add coconut milk and cocoa powder to pot and whisk. Once warmed, add chocolate and whisk.
9. Drain bacon bits on paper towel, reserving drippings. Add warm drippings to chocolate mixture. Whisk until chocolate melts and mixture emulsifies. Set bacon bits aside.
10. Remove pan from oven at let cool about 5 minutes. Then remove donuts from pan.
11. Ice donuts with chocolate sauce then sprinkle with bacon bits.
12. Transfer decorated donuts to serving dish.
13. Serve warm. Or let cool completely and serve room temperature.

NOTE: Bake in 8 mini cake pans or specialty cake pop pans lightly coated with coconut oil for fillable donuts or donut holes if you do not have a donut pan.

stevia, raw honey or agave nectar

Health Conscious Baking

Mocha Brownie Bites

Prep Time: 5 minutes

Cook Time: 25 minutes

Servings: 16

INGREDIENTS

4 cage-free eggs

1 cup cocoa powder

1/4 cup coconut oil

1/4 cup full-fat coconut milk

1/4 cup sweetener*

2 teaspoons instant espresso (or instant coffee)

1 teaspoon vanilla

INSTRUCTIONS

1. Preheat oven to 350 degrees F. Lightly oil square baking dish or line with parchment.
2. Add eggs, coconut oil, coconut milk and sweetener to medium mixing bowl and beat with hand mixer or whisk. Sift in cocoa powder, espresso and vanilla. Beat until well combined.
3. Pour batter into prepared baking pan and bake for 20 - 25 minutes, until set.
4. Allow to cool completely.
5. Slice and serve room temperature. Or refrigerate and serve chilled.

raw honey, agave nectar or maple syrup

Blueberry Scones

Prep Time: 5 minutes

Cook Time: 25 minutes

Servings: 8

INGREDIENTS

2 cups almond flour

1/3 cup arrowroot powder (or tapioca flour)

1 cage-free egg

1/2 cup dried or frozen blueberries

1/4 cup coconut oil

2 tablespoons sweetener*

2 teaspoons baking powder

1/2 teaspoon vanilla

1/2 teaspoon sea salt

1/4 teaspoon ground cinnamon (optional)

INSTRUCTIONS

1. Preheat oven to 350 degrees F. Line sheet pan with parchment or coat with coconut oil.
2. Whisk together almond flour, arrowroot powder, baking powder, salt, vanilla and cinnamon (optional) in medium mixing bowl.
3. In small mixing bowl, beat egg, oil and sweetener with hand mixer or whisk. Add egg mixture to dry ingredients and mix until well combined.

4. Fold in blueberries. Form dough into ball and place on sheet pan . Pat down to flatten to about 1/2 inch thick circle.
5. Cut into eight wedges with pizza cutter or sharp knife. Arrange at least 1 inch apart on sheet pan and bake for 20 - 25 minutes , or until edges are golden brown.
6. Remove from oven and let cool at least 10 minutes.
7. Serve room temperature.

Easy Poppy Seed Muffins

Prep Time: 5 minutes

Cook Time: 20 minutes

Servings: 12

INGREDIENTS

6 eggs

1/2 cup coconut flour

1/4 cup coconut oil

1/4 cup sweetener*

1 teaspoon vanilla

1 teaspoon poppy seeds

1/2 teaspoon baking soda

Juice of 2 lemons

Zest of 2 lemons

INSTRUCTIONS

1. Preheat oven to 350 degrees F. Oil muffin pan or line with paper liners.
2. Zest, *then* juice 2 lemons. Add to large mixing bowl with eggs, coconut oil, sweetener and vanilla. Beat with hand mixer or whisk until well combined.
3. Sift coconut flour and baking soda into wet ingredients, and mix until smooth. Stir in poppy seeds.
4. Use ice cream scoop or tablespoon to pour batter into prepared muffin pan.

5. Place in oven and bake for about 20 minutes, or until golden around edges and toothpick inserted into middle comes out clean.
6. Remove from oven and let cool for 5 minutes.
7. Serve warm. Or allow to cool completely and serve room temperature.

raw honey or agave nectar

Coconut Macaroons

Prep Time: 10 minutes

Cook Time: 20 minutes

Servings: 12

INGREDIENTS

6 cage-free egg whites

3 cups flaked coconut

1/2 cup sweetener*

1 tablespoon coconut oil

1 teaspoon vanilla

1/4 teaspoon sea salt

INSTRUCTIONS

1. Preheat oven to 350 degrees F. Line a sheet pan with parchment paper or baking mat.
2. In large mixing bowl, beat room temperature egg whites with hand mixer to stiff peaks, about 7 - 8 minutes.
3. Beat in sweetener, vanilla and salt until combined. Fold in 1 cup of coconut at a time.
4. Use ice cream scoop or spoon to drop rounds of batter onto prepared sheet pan.
5. Bake for about 20 minutes, or until coconut is toasted and browned.
6. Allow to cool on pan for 10 minutes. Then remove from pan.

7. Serve warm. Or allow to cool completely and serve room temperature.

* raw honey or agave nectar

Blackberry Dumplings

Prep Time: 15 minutes

Cook Time: 20 minutes

Servings: 8

INGREDIENTS

Blackberry Filling

2 1/2 cups blackberries (fresh or frozen)

2 - 4 tablespoons sweetener*

2 tablespoons tapioca flour

1/2 teaspoon ground black pepper

Zest of 1/2 lemon

Dumplings

1/4 cup coconut flour

3/4 cup almond flour

3 tablespoons cold coconut oil

1 teaspoon baking powder

1/2 teaspoon ground cinnamon

1/4 teaspoon sea salt

2 cage-free eggs

2 tablespoon sweetener

1 teaspoon vanilla

Zest of 1/2 lemon

INSTRUCTIONS

1. For *Dumplings*, sift coconut flour, almond flour, baking powder and salt into small mixing bowl. Cut in cold coconut oil with fork until crumbly. Place in freezer for 10 minutes.

2. Preheat oven to 400 degrees F.

3. For *Blackberry Filling*, add blackberries, sweetener, black pepper and lemon zest to medium pot. Heat over medium heat and bring to simmer. Whisk in tapioca flour and simmer about 10 minutes.

4. Pour hot blackberries into casserole dish and place in hot oven.

5. In medium bowl, beat eggs, sweetener, lemon zest, cinnamon and vanilla. Add chilled flour mixture to eggs and mix until dough comes together.

6. Carefully remove dish from oven and drop 8 dumplings onto bubbling berries.

7. Return dish to oven and bake 15 - 20 min, until dumplings are golden, set and cooked through.

8. Remove dish from oven and allow to cool about 5 minutes.

9. Serve warm. Or allow to cool completely and serve room temperature.

*stevia, raw honey or agave nectar

Carrot Cake Cookie Bars

Prep Time: 10 minutes

Cook Time: 25 minutes

Servings: 12

INGREDIENTS

2 cups almond meal

2 cups shredded carrots (about 4 large carrots)

3 cage-free eggs

1/4 cup coconut oil

1/2 cup unsweetened applesauce

1/2 cup flaked coconut

1/4 cup sweetener*

2 teaspoons vanilla

2 teaspoons ground cinnamon

1 teaspoon ground nutmeg

1/2 teaspoon ground black pepper

1/2 teaspoon sea salt

INSTRUCTIONS

1. Preheat oven to 350 Degrees F. Line baking pan with parchment or coat lightly with coconut oil.
2. Grate carrots, or process in food processor or bullet blender until finely chopped. Add to medium bowl.

3. Add eggs, oil, applesauce and sweetener to food processor or bullet blender. Process until thickened and light, about 1 - 2 minutes.

4. Pour egg mixture into carrots. Sift in almond flour and salt. Add vanilla and spices. Mix well with a wooden spoon or hand mixer. Stir in coconut.

5. Press dough evenly into prepared baking pan and bake about 25 minutes, or until firm and golden brown.

6. Remove from oven and allow to cool about 10 minutes.

7. Slice into bars and serve warm. Or let cool completely and serve room temperature.

*stevia, raw honey, agave nectar or maple syrup

Chocolate Zucchini Cake

Prep Time: 10 minutes

Cook Time: 25 minutes

Servings: 12

INGREDIENTS

1 1/2 cups almond flour

2 cage-free eggs

1 medium zucchini (1 1/2 cups grated)

1/2 cup unsweetened applesauce

1/4 cup coconut oil

1/4 - 1/2 cup sweetener*

1/4 cup cocoa powder

2 tablespoons ground chia seed (or flax meal)

1 teaspoon baking soda

1 teaspoon baking powder

1 teaspoon vanilla

1 teaspoon ground cinnamon

1 teaspoon ground black pepper

1/2 teaspoon sea salt

1/4 cup cocoa nibs or chocolate chips (optional)

INSTRUCTIONS

1. Preheat oven to 350 degrees F. Line rectangular baking pan with parchment or lightly coat with coconut oil.

2. Add eggs, coconut oil, applesauce and sweetener to food processor or bullet blender. Process until mixture is thick and lightened.
3. Grate zucchini and add to medium mixing bowl. Pour egg mixture over grated zucchini.
4. Sift almond flour, cocoa powder, chia meal, baking soda and powder, salt and spices into bowl. Beat with hand mixer or whisk to combine. Stir in cocoa nibs or chocolate chips (optional).
5. Pour batter into prepared baking pan and bake for about 25 minutes, until toothpick inserted into center comes out clean.
6. Remove from oven and let cool about 10 minutes.
7. Slice and serve warm. Or let cool completely and serve room temperature.

*stevia, raw honey or agave nectar

Cocoa Cream Muffins

Prep Time: 10 minutes*

Cook Time: 20 minutes

Servings: 12

INGREDIENTS

1 cup almond flour

1 cup coconut flour

3 cage-free eggs

1/2 cup unsweetened applesauce

1/4 cup coconut oil

1/4 cup sweetener*

1 avocado

3 tablespoons cocoa powder

1 tablespoon baking powder

1/4 teaspoon ground black pepper

1 teaspoon sea salt

Filling

2 cups water

1 cup cashews

3 tablespoons sweetener*

2 tablespoon cocoa powder

2 - 4 tablespoons coconut milk

INSTRUCTIONS

1. *Soak cashews overnight in 2 cups water. Drain and rinse. Set aside.

2. Preheat oven to 350 degrees F. Line muffin pan with paper liners or coat with coconut oil.

3. Slice avocado in half, pit, and scoop flesh into food processor or blender. Add eggs, coconut oil, applesauce and sweetener. Process until smooth.

4. Pour avocado blend into medium mixing bowl. Sift in almond flour, cocoa powder, baking powder, salt and pepper. Beat with hand mixer or whisk until combined.

5. Pour batter into prepared muffin pan. Bake 20 -25 minutes, or until firm but springy in center.

6. For *Filling*, add soaked cashews, sweetener and cocoa powder to food processor or bullet blender. Process until smooth and creamy. Add coconut milk if necessary to reach desired consistency.

7. Remove muffins from oven and let cool.

8. Scoop out center of muffin with knife or teaspoon, and fill with *Filling*. Or transfer *Filling* to pastry bag fitted with 1/2 inch tip, insert tip into muffin and fill.

9. Serve warm or room temperature.

*stevia, raw honey or agave nectar

Ginger Spice Cookies

Prep Time: 15 minutes

Cook Time: 15 minutes

Servings: 6

INGREDIENTS

1 1/2 cups almond flour

1 cage-free egg

1/4 cup sweetener*

2 tablespoons coconut oil

1 teaspoon ground chia seed (or flax meal)

1/4 teaspoon baking soda

1 tablespoon ground ginger

1/2 teaspoon ground clove

Pinch all spice

Pinch ground black pepper

Pinch sea salt

INSTRUCTIONS

1. Preheat oven to 350 degrees F. Line sheet pan with parchment or baking mat, or lightly coat with coconut oil.
2. Beat egg, oil, sweetener and chia meal in medium mixing bowl with hand mixer or whisk.
3. Add almond flour, baking soda, salt and spices. Mix until combined.
4. Chill batter in freezer for 5 - 10 minutes.

5. Scoop chilled batter into 6 large rounds on prepared sheet pan. Press into disk shape with hand.

6. Bake for about 15 minutes, until firm around the edges and golden brown.

7. Remove from oven and let cool about 10 minutes.

8. Serve warm. Or let cool completely and serve room temperature.

raw honey, agave nectar, grade B maple syrup, molasses

Lemon Coconut Bars

Prep Time: 15 minutes

Cook Time: 30 minutes

Servings: 12

INGREDIENTS

Crust

1/2 cup raw cashews

2/3 cup coconut flour

2 cage-free eggs

2 tablespoons coconut oil

2 tablespoons sweetener*

1 tablespoon flaked coconut

1 teaspoon fresh lemon juice

1/2 teaspoon baking soda

1/2 teaspoon vanilla

Filling

2 cage-free eggs

2 cage-free egg yolks

1 cup fresh lemon juice (about 6 lemons)

1/2 cup sweetener*

1/3 - 1/2 cup flaked coconut

2 tablespoons coconut flour

1 teaspoon lemon zest

INSTRUCTIONS

1. Preheat oven to 350 degrees F. Lightly coat rectangular baking dish with coconut oil, or line with parchment.

2. For *Crust*, add cashews and coconut to food processor or bullet blender and process until finely ground. Add remaining *Crust* ingredients to food processor and pulse until dough comes together.

3. Press dough into bottom of baking dish, and slightly up the sides. Dock crust with fork to prevent bubbling.

4. Place crust in oven and bake for 8 - 10 minutes.

5. For *Filling*, beat eggs, egg yolks, lemon juice, lemon zest and sweetener with hand mixer or whisk in medium bowl.

6. Sift in coconut flour and beat to combine. Let mixture sit for 5 minutes. Add flaked coconut and beat again to combine.

7. Pour *Filling* over par baked crust. Place in oven and bake 20 minutes, until center is set but still slightly jiggly.

8. Remove from oven and let cool for 20 minutes. Refrigerate about 20 minutes, until fully set and chilled.

9. Serve chilled or room temperature.

* *raw honey or agave nectar*

Cocoa Spice Pinwheel Cookies

Prep Time: 10 minutes

Cook Time: 20 minutes

Servings: 12

INGREDIENTS

2 cups almond flour

2 tablespoon sweetener*

1 egg

1 teaspoon vanilla

1/2 teaspoon baking powder

1/4 teaspoon sea salt

Filling

2 tablespoons cocoa powder

2 tablespoons sweetener*

2 teaspoons ground cinnamon

1 teaspoon ground black pepper

1/2 teaspoon vanilla

INSTRUCTIONS

1. Preheat oven to 300 degrees F. Line sheet pan with parchment or baking mat. Prepare 2 additional sheets of parchment.
2. Add flour, egg, sweetener, vanilla, baking powder and salt to medium bowl. Blend with wooden spoon, then knead with hand to form thick dough.

3. Divide dough in half. Place half of dough in small mixing bowl. Add all *Filling* ingredients to bowl and mix until well combined.
4. Roll out each half of dough separately on parchment sheets. Roll into equal rectangles.
5. Place *Filling* rectangle on top of plain dough. Use parchment to help roll dough tightly along long edge into log.
6. Use sharp knife to cut log into 1/4 round slices. Place cookies on prepared sheet pan and bake about 10 minutes, until edges are golden brown.
7. Remove from oven and let cool about 5 minutes.
8. Serve warm. Or let cool completely and serve room temperature.

*raw honey, agave nectar or maple syrup

Rosemary Basil Scones

Prep Time: 10 minutes

Cook Time: 25 minutes

Servings: 8

INGREDIENTS

2 cups almond flour

1/3 cup arrowroot flour

1 egg

1/4 cup organic coconut oil

1/2 lemon

2 tablespoons sweetener*

2 teaspoons baking powder

2 sprigs fresh rosemary

 5 - 6 large basil leaves (or 1 1/2 teaspoons dried basil)

1/2 teaspoon vanilla

1/2 teaspoon sea salt

1/4 cup hazelnuts (optional)

INSTRUCTIONS

1. Preheat oven to 350 degrees F. Line sheet pan with parchment
   or coat with coconut oil.

2. Whisk together flours, baking powder, salt and vanilla in large
   mixing bowl.

3. Zest 1/2 lemon into small mixing bowl. Finely chop rosemary
   and chiffon fresh basil. Add herbs to bowl with egg and

sweetener. Beat with hand mixer or whisk while slowly pouring in coconut oil.

4. Add egg mixture to flour blend and mix until well combined.

5. Chop and fold in hazelnuts (optional). Form dough into ball and place on sheet pan. Flatten to 1/2 inch thick circle with hands.

6. Cut into eight wedges with pizza cutter or sharp knife. Arrange at least 1 inch apart on sheet pan and bake for 20 - 25 minutes , or until edges are golden brown.

7. Remove and let cool. Serve room temperature.

orange juice, raw honey, agave nectar or maple syrup

Cinnamon Rolls

Prep Time: 10 minutes

Cook Time: 20 minutes

Servings: 8

INGREDIENTS

Dough

3 cups almond flour

3 eggs

1/2 cup dried pitted dates

1/4 cup ground chia seed (or flax meal)

1/4 cup tapioca flour (or arrowroot powder)

1/4 cup nut milk

2 teaspoons baking powder

1/4 teaspoon sea salt

Topping

1/2 cup dried pitted dates

1/2 cup full-fat coconut milk

Filling

2 tablespoons melted cacao butter (coconut oil)

1/2 cup dried pitted dates

2 tablespoons ground cinnamon

INSTRUCTIONS

1. Preheat oven to 350 degrees F. Line muffin pan with paper liners or coat with coconut oil. Cover cutting board with parchment and coat heavily with coconut oil.
2. For *Dough*, heat nut milk in small pan over medium heat. Whisk in tapioca until combined. Remove from heat.
3. Add dates and eggs to food processor or high-speed blender. Process until thick, light mixture forms.
4. Add date mixture and tapioca mixture to medium mixing bowl. Beat in chia meal, baking soda, salt and almond flour 1 cup at a time with hand mixer or whisk.
5. Place dough on prepared parchment. Oil hands to prevent sticking and press dough into 1/2 inch thick rectangle.
6. For *Filling*, place all ingredients in clean food processor or high-speed blender and process until finely ground or smooth.
7. Roll dough into log along edge using parchment paper. Use sharp knife or floss to slice log into rolls. Place in muffin pan.
8. For *Topping*, place dates and coconut milk in clean food processor or high-speed blender and process until smooth and creamy. Pour over rolls in muffin pan.
9. Place in oven and bake about 20 minutes, or until cinnamon bubbles and dough is firm.
10. Remove from oven and let cool at least 5 minutes.
11. Serve immediately. Or let cool completely and serve room temperature.

NOTE: Bake in oiled round baking dish or cake pan for 30 - 35 minutes for **Pan Cinnamon Rolls**.

Coconut Baked Donut

Prep Time: 5 minutes

Cook Time: 20 minutes

Servings: 6

INGREDIENTS

Donuts

1 3/4 cups almond flour

1 tablespoon coconut flour

2 eggs

1/3 cup coconut oil

1/4 cup unsweetened applesauce

1/4 cup sweetener*

2 tablespoons nut milk

2 teaspoons vanilla

3/4 teaspoon baking soda

1/2 teaspoon sea salt

Topping

1/2 cup flaked or shredded coconut

1/4 cup full-fat coconut milk

2 tablespoon sweetener

1/4 teaspoon vanilla

INSTRUCTIONS

1. Preheat oven to 350 degreesF. Lightly coat donut pan with coconut oil.
2. Add almond and coconut flours, baking soda and salt to food processor or high-speed blender. Process for 1 minute.
3. Add eggs, sweetener, coconut oil, applesauce, nut milk and vanilla. Process until light, thick batter forms, about 1 - 2 minutes.
4. Pour batter into donut pan until wells are 3/4 full.
5. Place in oven and bake for about 20 minutes, until dough is set and lightly browned.
6. For *Topping*, combine coconut milk, sweetener and vanilla in small mixing bowl.
7. Remove pan from oven at let cool about 5 minutes. Then remove donuts from pan.
8. Dip donuts in coconut icing then sprinkle with flaked or shredded coconut.
9. Transfer decorated donuts to serving dish.
10. Serve warm. Or let cool completely and serve room temperature.

NOTE: Bake in 8 mini cake pans or specialty cake pop pans lightly coated with coconut oil for fillable donuts or donut holes if you do not have a donut pan.

* stevia, raw honey or agave nectar

Blueberry Lavender Blondies

Prep Time: 10 minutes

Cook Time: 30 minutes

Servings: 12

INGREDIENTS

4 eggs

3/4 cup coconut flour

2 tablespoons arrowroot powder (or tapioca flour)

1 cup (1/2 pint) fresh blueberries

1/2 cup sweetener*

1/4 cup full-fat coconut milk

1/2 teaspoon baking powder

2 teaspoons vanilla

1 teaspoon food-grade lavender buds (ground)

1/2 teaspoon sea salt

INSTRUCTIONS
1. Preheat oven to 350 degrees F. Coat rectangular baking pan or "all-corner" specialty brownie pan with coconut oil.
2. Add blueberries to food processor or bullet blender with coconut milk and process until smooth. Set aside.
3. Beat eggs in medium mixing bowl with hand mixer or whisk. Add blueberry purée, sweetener, vanilla and lavender. Mix to combine.
4. Sift coconut flour, arrowroot or tapioca, baking powder and salt into blueberry mixture. Beat until well combined.

5. Scrape batter into prepared baking pan and smooth top with spatula.

6. Bake for 25 - 30 minutes, until center is firm and top is golden brown. Toothpick inserted into center will come out moist but mostly clean.

7. Remove from oven and allow to cool about 10 minutes.

8. Slice and serve warm. Or allow to cool completely and serve room temperature.

*stevia, raw honey or agave nectar

Savory Spiced Pineapple Bread

Prep Time: 5 minutes

Cook Time: 20 minutes

Servings: 8

INGREDIENTS

2 cups almond flour

3 eggs

1/4 cup coconut oil

1 cup crushed pineapple (canned in juice or fresh)

1 tablespoon apple cider vinegar

2 teaspoons baking soda

2 teaspoons vanilla

2 teaspoons ground cinnamon

2 teaspoons ground ginger

1/2 teaspoon ground nutmeg

1/2 teaspoon paprika

1/2 teaspoon cayenne pepper

1 teaspoon ground white pepper (or black pepper)

1 teaspoon sea salt

1 teaspoon cardamom (optional)

1 teaspoon turmeric (optional)

INSTRUCTIONS

1. Preheat oven to 350 degrees F. Coat 2 small loaf pans with coconut oil.

2. Separate eggs. In large bowl, beats egg whites to soft peaks with hand mixer or whisk, about 5 minutes. Add yolks, crushed or blended pineapple, coconut oil and vinegar. Beat well.
3. In medium bowl, blend flour, baking soda, spices and salt. Pour flour mixture into egg mixture and mix well.
4. Pour batter into loaf pans and bake for about 25 minutes, until toothpick inserted into center comes out clean.
5. Remove oven and let cool at least 5 minutes. Insert knife around edges and remove from pan.
6. Slice and serve warm. Or let cool completely and serve room temperature.

NOTE: Bake in large oiled loaf pan for 35 - 45 minutes for **Savory Spiced Pineapple Loaf**.

Strawberry Bread

Prep Time: 10 minutes

Cook Time: 10 minutes

Servings: 12 - 16

INGREDIENTS

1 cup coconut flour

3/4 cup cashew flour (or almond flour)

1/4 cup ground chia seed (or flax meal)

1/2 cup coconut oil

2 eggs

1/4 cup coconut crème

1/4 cup sweetener*

1/4 cup unsweetened apple sauce

1 teaspoons baking powder

1 tablespoon ground cinnamon

1 teaspoon ground ginger

1 teaspoon ground white pepper (or black pepper)

1 teaspoon sea salt

2 cups fresh sliced strawberries

1/2 cup chopped walnuts (optional)

INSTRUCTIONS

1. Preheat oven to 350 degrees F. Line muffin pan with paper liners or coat with coconut oil.

2. In large bowl, whisk eggs with hand mixer or whisk until frothy and light. Add coconut oil, sweetener and applesauce. Blend until combined. Slice strawberries, and fold in with walnuts (optional).

3. In medium bowl, blend flours, chia meal, baking powder, salt and spices. Stir flour blend into strawberry mixture until well combined.

4. Use ice cream scoop or tablespoon to scoop equal portions of batter into muffin pans, 1/2 - 3/4 full. Line or oil more muffin pans if excess batter remains.

5. Bake for 15 minutes, or until golden brown and firm but springy to the touch.

6. Cool enough to handle. Serve warm or room temperature.

NOTE: Bake in square oiled baking pan for 25 - 35 minutes or two oiled loaf pans for 35 - 45 minutes for **Strawberry Loaves**.

stevia, raw honey or agave nectar

Apple Cider Bread

Prep Time: 10 minutes

Cook Time: 20 minutes

Servings: 24

INGREDIENTS

2 cups coconut flour

1 cup almond flour

12 ounces organic hard cider

2 eggs

1/2 cup unsweetened applesauce

1 tart apple

2 tablespoons baking powder

1 teaspoon ground nutmeg

1 teaspoon ground black pepper

1 teaspoon sea salt

INSTRUCTIONS

1. Preheat oven to 375 degrees F. Line 2 muffin pans with paper liners or coat with coconut oil.
2. Peel, core and grate or dice apple, and place in large bowl. Pour hard apple cider over apples, plus nutmeg and black pepper.
3. In medium bowl, whisk eggs with hand mixer or whisk until frothy and light. Add applesauce and blend until combined. Add egg mixture to cider and apples.

4. Slowly sift and stir flours, baking powder and salt into wet ingredients.

5. Use ice cream scoop or tablespoon to scoop equal portions of batter into muffin pans, 1/2 - 3/4 full.

6. Bake for 15 - 20 minutes, or until golden brown and firm but springy to the touch.

7. Cool enough to handle. Serve warm or room temperature.

NOTE: Bake in square oiled baking pan for 35 - 45 minutes or two oiled loaf pans for 45 - 55 minutes for **Apple Cider Loaves**.

stevia, raw honey or agave nectar

No Corn "Corn" Muffins

Prep Time: 5 minutes

Cook Time: 15 minutes

Servings: 12

INGREDIENTS

1 cup almond flour

2 eggs

1/4 cup coconut oil

2 tablespoons unsweetened applesauce

1 teaspoon sweetener*

1 teaspoon organic apple cider vinegar

1 teaspoon baking powder

1/2 teaspoon ground turmeric (optional)

Pinch ground white pepper (optional)

INSTRUCTIONS

1. Preheat oven to 350 degrees F. Line muffin pan with paper liners or lightly coat with coconut oil.

2. Beat eggs in medium mixing bowl with hand mixer or whisk until thick and slightly frothy. Add oil, applesauce, sweetener, and vinegar and mix well.

3. Stir in almond meal, baking powder, and turmeric and white pepper (optional) until combined.

4. Use ice cream scoop or tablespoon to scoop batter into muffin pan, about 1/2 - 3/4 full.

5. Bake 15 - 18 minutes until edges are golden brown and the tops are firm.

6. Serve warm or room temperature.

NOTE: Bake in square oiled baking pan for 25 - 35 minutes for **"Corn"** **Bread**.

stevia, raw honey or agave nectar

English Muffins

Prep Time: 5 minutes

Cook Time: 15 minutes

Servings: 4

INGREDIENTS

1/3 cup coconut flour

4 eggs

1/4 cup almond milk (or low-fat coconut milk)

2 tablespoons coconut oil

1 tablespoon unsweetened applesauce

1/2 teaspoon baking soda

1 teaspoon organic apple cider vinegar

Pinch sea salt

INSTRUCTIONS

1. Preheat oven to 400 degrees F. Coat 4 mini-round cake pans or 4-inch diameter oven safe ramekins with coconut oil.
2. In small mixing bowl mix baking soda and apple cider vinegar together. Set aside and allow to froth.
3. In medium bowl, beat eggs with hand mixer or whisk until thick and frothy. Add flour, milk, applesauce and salt. Combine.
4. Add baking soda and vinegar mixture and blend well until smooth and free of clumps.
5. Pour batter into pans or ramekins and bake for 12 - 15 minutes, until slightly golden and center is firm to the touch.

6. Remove muffins from oven. Loosen from sides of pan or container with knife turn out.
7. Serve warm. Muffins will have traditional **English Crumpet** texture.

NOTE: For crusty, American style **English Muffins**, cut in half and toast in skillet coated with coconut oil. Press muffin down in pan with spatula and flip, browning on both sides.

stevia, raw honey or agave nectar

Easy Pita

Prep Time: 5 minutes

Cook Time: 20 minutes

Servings: 1

INGREDIENTS

1 cup tapioca flour/starch

1 egg

2 tablespoons coconut oil (or almond oil)

1 teaspoon ground chia seed (flax meal)

5 tablespoons water

1/2 teaspoon baking soda

1/4 teaspoon sea salt

INSTRUCTIONS

1. Preheat oven to 375 degrees F. Cover sheet pan with parchment paper. Heat small pot over low heat.

2. Mix 1/3 cup flour, chia meal, water and 1 tablespoon oil in pan. Stir until mixture comes together. Remove from heat and cool in freezer.

3. In medium bowl, blend remaining flour, baking soda and salt. Then add egg and remaining oil. Mix until combined .

4. Add cooled chia mixture to bowl. Mix to combine, then remove and knead to form dough.

5. Form round disk, then flatten on baking sheet lined with parchment.

6. Bake about 15 minutes. Carefully turn over with spatula and bake another 5 - 10 minutes, or until crisp.

7. Remove from oven and cut into wedges. Serve warm or cooled.

NOTE: For **Pita Chips** , place baked wedges on oiled sheet pan, brush tops with coconut oil and broil in oven for about 2 minutes on each side. *Watch carefully and do not burn!*

Coconut Crisps

Prep Time: 10 minutes

Cook Time: 10 minutes

Servings: 4

INGREDIENTS

1 cup coconut flour

3/4 cup almond flour

4 egg whites

1/4 cup coconut oil

1/4 cup coconut crème

1/4 cup sweetener

1/2 cup flaked coconut

1 teaspoon vanilla

1/2 teaspoon baking soda

3/4 teaspoon sea salt

1/2 teaspoon ground white pepper (or black pepper)

INSTRUCTIONS

1. Preheat oven to 375 degrees F. Line sheet pan with parchment paper or coat with coconut oil. Prepare two additional sheets of parchment.

2. Whisk egg and oil with hand mixer or whisk until blended and slightly frothy. Add sweetener, coconut crème and vanilla, and continue blending.

3. Sift in half of flour, baking soda, vanilla, salt and pepper. Add coconut flakes. Sift in remaining flour. Stir and bring dough together.
4. Form dough into rectangle and flatten with hands on parchment. Cover with second sheet of parchment and flatten to about 1/4 inch with rolling pin. Remove top layer of parchment.
5. Cut rectangles from dough with pizza cutter or sharp knife. Carefully flip dough onto sheet pan. Arrange at least 1/2 inch apart on sheet pan.
6. Bake for about 10 minutes, or until crisp and golden brown. Remove and let cool. Serve room temperature.

Angel Food Cake

Prep Time: 15 minutes

Cook Time: 30 minutes

Servings: 12

INGREDIENTS

12 egg whites (room temperature)

1/2 cup sweetener*

3/4 cup arrowroot powder

1/4 cup coconut flour

1 1/2 teaspoons cream of tartar (optional)

1 teaspoon baking soda

1 1/2 teaspoons vanilla

1/4 teaspoon sea salt

INSTRUCTIONS

1. Preheat oven to 325 degrees F.
2. Sift arrowroot and coconut flour into small mixing bowl. Set aside.
3. In large mixing bowl, beat egg whites until they foam. Add baking soda, salt, vanilla and cream of tartar (optional). Beat egg whites well into soft peaks, about 5 minutes. Slowly drizzle in sweetener while beating to just under stiff peaks.
4. Gently fold four mixture into the egg whites with spatula.

5. Spoon batter into 6 - 8 ungreased mini tube or Bundt® pans. Use butter knife to cut through batter and make sure batter settles well into pans, then smooth tops.

6. Place pan on sheet pan and bake 20 - 25 minutes, or until top is golden brown and firm but springy.

7. Remove from oven and invert pans onto small raisers, like a butter knife or other small heatsafe object. This helps prevent the cakes from collapsing. Allow to cool completely

8. Serve room temperature.

raw honey or agave nectar

NOTE: Bake in Angel Food pan or tube pan for 1 hour for large **Angel Food Cake**.

Chocolate Mint Milano Cookies

Prep Time: 30 minutes

Cook Time: 15 minutes

Servings: 12

INGREDIENTS

Cocoa Lady Fingers

1/3 cup coconut flour

3 tablespoons arrowroot powder

4 eggs

1/4 cup sweetener*

2 tablespoons cocoa powder

1/2 teaspoon baking powder

1/2 teaspoon vanilla

Mint Chocolate Filling

4 oz organic dark chocolate

2 oz full-fat coconut milk

4 drops pure mint extract/oil

INSTRUCTIONS

1. Preheat oven to 400 degrees F. Line two sheet pans with parchment paper. Fit pastry bag with 1/2 inch round tip, or cut 1/4 inch corner off sturdy kitchen storage bag (like Ziploc®).

2. For *Cocoa Lady Fingers*, beat egg yolks, sweetener and vanilla until thick and pale.

3. In separate bowl, beat egg whites to stiff peaks with hand mixer or whisk, about 8 minutes.

4. Fold half of egg whites into egg yolk mixture. Then sift in coconut flour, cocoa, arrowroot powder and baking powder. Gently fold batter. Fold in remaining egg whites until mixture is uniform.

5. Scoop batter into pastry or storage bag. Place in tall round container and fold open end of bag over edge of container for easier prep.

6. Pipe 4 inch cookies onto prepared sheet pans about 2 inches apart.

7. Place in oven and bake for 8 minutes, until set and just golden.

8. Remove cookies from oven and transfer full parchment sheet onto wire rack to cool completely. Do not try to remove warm cookies from parchment.

9. Heat 1 inch of water in bottom of double boiler, or in bottom pan with metal or glass bowl on top.

10. For *Mint Chocolate Filling*, melt chocolate and coconut milk over double boiler until smooth. Remove from heat and stir in mint extract/oil.

11. Remove cooled *Cocoa Lady Fingers* from parchment. Dip bottom of cookie into chocolate mint mixture and press against bottom of second cookie to make sandwich. Repeat with remaining cookies.

12. Serve warm. Or let chocolate set for 10 minutes, in refrigerator if preferred, and serve chilled or room temperature.

*stevia, raw honey or agave nectar

Easy Lunch Recipes

Soft Baked Pita

Prep Time: 5 minutes

Cook Time: 20 minutes

Servings: 1

INGREDIENTS

1 cup tapioca flour

1 tablespoon ground chia seed (or flax meal)

2 eggs

2 tablespoons coconut oil

1/4 cup water

1/2 teaspoon baking soda

1/4 teaspoon sea salt

INSTRUCTIONS

1. Preheat oven to 350 degrees F. Cover sheet pan with parchment paper or baking mat. Heat small pot over low heat.
2. Mix 1/3 cup tapioca flour with chia meal, water and 1 tablespoon coconut oil in pot. Stir until mixture comes together. Remove from heat and cool in freezer.
3. In medium bowl, blend remaining tapioca flour, baking soda and salt. Then beat in eggs and remaining oil with hand mixer or whisk until combined.
4. Add cooled chia mixture to egg mixture and mix to combine with wooden spoon or spatula. Remove mixture and knead to form soft dough.

5. Form large round disk and flatten on lined baking sheet with hands or rolling pin.

6. Place in oven and bake for about 10 minutes. Carefully turn over with spatula and bake another 10 minutes, or until firm.

7. Remove from oven and let cool about 5 minutes.

8. Fill with grilled meats and veggies and serve warm.

Cheese Steak Sandwich

Prep Time: 15 minutes*

Cook Time: 25 minutes

Servings: 4

INGREDIENTS

Sandwich Bread

1 cup tapioca flour/starch

1/4 - 1/3 cup coconut flour

1 egg

1/2 cup warm water

1/4 cup coconut oil

1/4 cup applesauce

1 teaspoon apple cider vinegar

1/2 teaspoon baking soda

1 teaspoon sea salt

Almond Cheese

1 cup skinless almonds*

2 tablespoons coconut oil (or walnut oil)

1 tablespoons lemon juice

1 tablespoon apple cider vinegar

1 garlic clove

1/4 teaspoon ground white pepper (or black pepper)

1/2 teaspoon sea salt

1/4 cup water

Filling

8 oz beef steak

1 small onion

1/2 bell pepper

1/2 teaspoon ground black pepper

1/2 teaspoon Sea salt

INSTRUCTIONS

1. *Soak almonds in enough water to cover overnight. Drain and rinse.
2. Preheat oven to 350 degrees F. Line sheet pan with parchment paper or coat with coconut oil.
3. In medium bowl, sift together tapioca flour, 1/4 cup coconut flour, baking soda and salt. Stir in warm water and oil.
4. Whisk egg in small bowl. Add applesauce and vinegar. Add egg mixture to flour mixture and mix until well combined. Add 1 tablespoon coconut flour or water at a time if needed to form soft and slightly sticky dough.
5. Divide dough into 3 portions and roll into loaves. Dust your hand with extra tapioca flour to prevent sticking.
6. Place loaves on sheet pan and pat down slightly. Bake 20 - 25minutes, or until edges are golden brown and the tops are firm. Remove from oven and allow to cool.
7. While *Sandwich Bread* is baking, add all *Almond Cheese* ingredients to food processor or bullet blender and process until

smooth. Add 1 tablespoon of water at a time to reach preferred consistency.

8. Heat medium skillet over medium-high heat. Add 1 tablespoon coconut oil to hot pan.

9. Thinly slice steak, onion and pepper. Add steak to hot pan and sauté about 1 minute. Add veggies, salt and pepper. Sauté about 5 minutes, until meat is cooked and veggies are soft and caramelized. Remove from heat and set aside.

10. Slice cooled *Sandwich Bread* in half and spread on *Almond Cheese*. Layer meat and veggies on bread.

11. Serve immediately. Or wrap in plastic wrap or parchment and store in lidded container.

Asian Empanada

Prep Time: 20 minutes

Cook Time: 20 minutes

Servings: 4

INSTRUCTIONS

Crust

1 cup almond flour

1 cup coconut flour

2 eggs

3 tablespoons sesame oil (or coconut oil)

1/2 teaspoon garlic powder

1/2 teaspoon onion powder

1/2 teaspoon ground ginger

1/4 teaspoon baking soda

1 teaspoon sea salt

1 tablespoon sesame oil (or coconut oil)

1 tablespoon sesame seeds

Filling

6 oz chicken or shrimp

1/2 head cabbage (1 cup shredded)

1 carrot

1/4 cup mushrooms

2 inch piece fresh ginger

2 garlic cloves

1 tablespoon pure fish sauce

1 teaspoon apple cider vinegar

1 shallot

1 scallion

1 teaspoon sesame oil

DIRECTIONS

1. For *Crust*, sift almond and coconut flour into medium mixing bowl. Add baking soda, spices and salt.
2. Whisk eggs in small mixing bowl, then add to flour and combine. Slowly add 3 tablespoons oil until malleable dough comes together.
3. Roll in plastic wrap or wrap tightly in parchment and refrigerate for 15 minutes.
4. Preheat oven to 400 degrees. Line sheet pan with parchment or baking mat. Cover cutting board with parchment. Het medium pan over medium heat.
5. Shred cabbage, grate carrot, slice mushrooms. Peel and grate ginger. Slice scallion. Peel and mince shallot and garlic. Dice chicken or slice shrimp in half.
6. Add sesame oil to pan. Add chicken or shrimp hot oiled pan with ginger, shallot and garlic. Sauté about 90 seconds. Add cabbage, carrot, and mushrooms and sauté for a minute.
7. Add vinegar and fish sauce. Sauté about 3 minutes until cabbage is wilted. Stir in scallions. Remove from heat and set aside.

8. Remove dough from refrigerator. Divide dough into 4 portions. Roll dough into balls and flatten on parchment covered cutting board with hands. Roll into circles about 1/8 inch thick with rolling pin.

9. Scoop equal portions of *Filling* into center of one side of dough circle. Fold bare half of dough over filled half. Press edges together, letting any trapped air escape. Crimp edges of dough together with fork. Repeat with remaining dough.

10. Bruch tops of empanada with sesame oil and sprinkle with sesame seeds.

11. Arrange empanadas on lined sheet pan and bake 15 - 20 minutes, or until dough is golden and cooked through.

12. Serve immediately. Or allow to cool and store in air-tight container.

Turkey Tenders

Prep Time: 5 minutes

Cook Time: 15 minutes

Servings: 2

INGREDIENTS

8 oz boneless skinless turkey

1 egg

1/2 cup almond meal

1 teaspoon flax meal

1/4 teaspoon garlic powder

1/2 teaspoon paprika

1/2 teaspoon ground sage

1/2 teaspoon ground black pepper

1/2 teaspoon sea salt

Cranberry Compote

1/4 cup dried cranberries

1 teaspoon sweetener*

1/2 teaspoon arrowroot powder (or tapioca flour)

1/2 cup water

INSTRUCTIONS

1. Heat a medium skillet over medium high heat. Lightly coat pan with coconut oil. Heat small pot over medium heat. Add 1/2 cup water and bring to boil.

2. Slice turkey into 1 inch wide strips. Arrange slices between 2 sheets of parchment and pound with kitchen mallet or rolling pin to flatten slightly. Place turkey between two paper towels to absorb excess moisture.
3. Blend almond meal, flax meal, spices and salt in a shallow dish.
4. Beat egg in small mixing bowl. Dip turkey strips into beaten egg, then dredge in seasoned almond meal.
5. Carefully place coated turkey into hot oil and fry about 3 - 4 minutes, until golden brown and cooked through. Turn half way through cooking with tongs.
6. Add cranberries to boiling water, and whisk in sweetener and arrowroot or tapioca. Reduce heat to medium and stir occasionally as compote thickens, about 5 - 8 minutes.
7. Drain cooked turkey on paper towel, then transfer to serving dish. Serve warm.
8. Or allow to cool and transfer to lidded container. Serve room temperature or chilled.
9. Pour *Cranberry Compote* into small serving bowl or lidded container. Serve with chicken.

stevia, raw honey or agave nectar

Soft Baked Pretzel

Prep Time: 15 minutes

Cook Time: 20 minutes

Servings: 4

INGREDIENTS

1 cup coconut flour

1/2 cup tapioca flour/starch

1/2 cup coconut oil

1/2 cup water

1 egg

2 tablespoon apple cider vinegar

1/2 teaspoon baking soda

1/2 teaspoon baking powder

1/2 teaspoon sea salt

INSTRUCTIONS

1. Preheat oven to 350 degrees F. Heat medium pan over medium-high heat. Line sheet pan with parchment or baking mat.

2. Add coconut oil, water, vinegar and salt to pot. Bring to a boil and remove from heat.

3. Whisk in tapioca flour. Stir with wooden spoon or soft spatula until mixture gels and comes together.

4. Stir in baking soda and baking powder. Continue mixing for a minute. Mixture will foam and expand. Let mixture sit and cool about 5 minutes.
5. Sift in coconut flour. Mix partially, then beat in egg. Blend until combined. Excess coconut flour may sit in bottom of bowl.
6. Turn out dough onto cutting board dusted with any excess coconut flour from mixture. Knead dough for 2 minutes.
7. Cut dough into 4 equal portions. Roll out pieces into ropes and twist to form classic pretzel twist. Pinch together any crumbled dough.
8. Arrange pretzels on lined sheet pan. Brush with coconut oil or full-fat coconut milk and sprinkle with salt.
9. Place sheet pan in oven and bake about 25 minutes, until cooked through.
10. Serve immediately with organic mustard. Or allow to cool and serve room temperature.

Frontier Anzac Biscuits

Prep Time: 5 minutes

Cook Time: 25 minutes

Servings: 4

INGREDIENTS

3/4 cup almond flour

3/4 cup sliced almonds

3/4 cup coconut flakes

1/4 cup sweetener*

1/4 cup coconut oil

1/2 teaspoon baking soda

1 tablespoon water

INSTRUCTIONS

1. Preheat oven to 300 degrees F. Line sheet pan with parchment sheet or baking mat.

2. In medium mixing bowl, combine almond flour, sliced almonds and coconut flakes.

3. Mix baking soda and water in small mixing bowl. Add to medium mixing bowl with sweetener and oil. Mix until combined. Add water 1 tablespoon at a time if dough is too crumbly.

4. Form 12 large biscuits and arrange on sheet pan. Flatten slightly with hand for even baking.

5. Bake for 25 - 30 minutes, until golden.

6. Serve immediately. Or allow to cool completely and pack in airtight container or sealable baggie.

raw honey or agave nectar

Raw Cashew Avocado Hummus

Prep Time: 5 minutes*

Servings: 4

INGREDIENTS

1 cup raw cashews

1 avocado

Juice of 1/2 lemon

2 garlic cloves

1 teaspoon ground white pepper (or black pepper)

1/2 teaspoon sea salt

INSTRUCTIONS

1. *Soak cashews in enough water to cover at least 4 hours. Drain and rinse.
2. Add soaked cashews to food processor or bullet blender with lemon juice, peeled garlic, salt and pepper. Process until smooth. Add water 1 tablespoon at a time if desired to reach thick, slightly grainy consistency.
3. Transfer cashew mixture to small mixing bowl. Cut avocado in half and remove pit. Scoop flesh into bowl and mash cashews and avocado together with fork.
4. Serve immediately. Or place in refrigerator and serve chilled.

Zucchini Salad with Sundried Tomato Sauce

Prep Time: 20 minutes*

Servings: 2

INGREDIENTS

1 medium zucchini

1 tomato

5 sundried tomatoes

1 garlic clove

2 fresh basil leaves

1 tablespoon raw virgin coconut oil (or 2 tablespoons warm water)

1/4 teaspoon ground white pepper (or black pepper)

1/4 teaspoon sea salt

INSTRUCTIONS

1. Run zucchini through spiralizer, slice into long, thin shreds with knife, or use vegetable peeler to make flat, thin slices. Sprinkle with a pinch of salt and pepper, and gently toss to coat.

2. Add tomato, sundried tomatoes, peeled garlic, basil, coconut oil or warm water, and remaining salt and pepper to food processor or bullet blender. Process until sauce of desired consistency forms.

3. Transfer zucchini pasta to serving bowls. Top with tomato sauce and serve immediately.
4. Or refrigerate for 20 minutes and serve chilled.

Spicy Tuna Tartare

Prep Time: 15* minutes

Servings: 4

INGREDIENTS

1 lb tuna steak (sushi grade)

1 small cucumber

1 ripe avocado

1 lime

1 garlic clove

1 hot chile pepper

2 tablespoons raw virgin coconut oil

Small bunch fresh cilantro

1 teaspoon red pepper flake

1 teaspoon sea salt

INSTRUCTIONS

1. Peel, seed and dice cucumber and avocado. Finely chop cilantro. Add to medium mixing bowl.
2. Remove seeds, stem and veins from hot pepper. Peel garlic and add to food processor or bullet blender with cayenne and hot pepper. Process until smooth paste forms. Add to bowl.
3. Dice tuna, discarding any tough white gristle. Add to bowl.
4. Squeeze on lime juice and add salt.
5. Gently toss with soft spatula or large spoon.
6. Serve immediately. Or refrigerate 20 minutes and serve chilled.

Spinach Mushroom Muffins

Prep Time: 10 minutes

Cook Time: 15 minutes

Servings: 12

INGREDIENTS

1 cup almond flour

2 eggs

1 cup fresh spinach

1/2 cup fresh mushrooms

1 tablespoon sweetener*

1 tablespoon apple cider vinegar

1 teaspoon baking soda

1 teaspoon baking powder

1 teaspoon ground white pepper (or black pepper)

1/2 teaspoon ground nutmeg

1/2 teaspoon dried basil

INSTRUCTIONS

1. Preheat oven to 350 degrees F. Line muffin pan with paper liners
   or lightly coat with coconut oil. Heat medium pan over medium-
   high heat.

2. Slice mushrooms and add to hot pan. Sauté about 3 minutes, then
   add spinach. Sauté until water evaporates, mushrooms are cooked
   through and spinach is wilted. Set aside.

3. Beat eggs, sweetener and vinegar in medium mixing bowl with hand mixer or whisk until thick and frothy.
4. Add sautéed veggies, almond flour, baking soda and powder and spices and mix until combined.
5. Use ice cream scoop or tablespoon to pour batter into prepared muffin pan.
6. Bake 15 - 20 minutes, until edges are golden brown and tops are firm.
7. Remove muffins from oven and let cool about 5 minutes.
8. Serve warm. Or allow to cool complete and serve temperature.

NOTE: Bake in square oiled baking pan for 30 - 35 minutes for **Spinach Mushroom Bread**.

stevia, raw honey or agave nectar

Pigs In A Blanket

Prep Time: 20 minutes

Cook Time: 15 minutes

Servings: 4

INGREDIENTS

1 package(26 count) nitrate-free/nitrite-free mini hot dogs

3 egg whites

1/4 cup almond flour

1/4 cup coconut flour

1 tablespoon cold coconut oil

1/2 teaspoon baking powder

Pinch garlic powder

Pinch sea salt

2 oz organic mustard

INSTRUCTIONS

1. In separate medium bowl, mix almond and coconut flours with baking powder. Cut-in cold coconut oil, then add pinch of garlic powder and salt. Mixture should be crumbly. Refrigerate 15 - 20 minutes.

2. Preheat oven to 400 degrees F. Line sheet pan with parchment or lightly coat with coconut oil.

3. Whisk egg whites in medium bowl until white and frothy, just before soft peaks develop.

4. Gently fold egg whites into refrigerated flour mixture until just combined.

5. Flatten 1 level teaspoon of dough into a rectangle in your fingers. Place one sausage in middle of dough wrap it around the sausage. Repeat with remaining sausage and dough.

6. Place wrapped sausages on prepared sheet pan and bake about 15 minutes, until dough is golden brown and links are heated through.

7. Serve hot with mustard.

Mighty Beef Sliders

Prep Time: 15 minutes

Cook Time: 25 minutes

Servings: 4

INGREDIENTS

Mini Burger Buns

1 1/2 cup raw cashews

1/3 cup coconut flour

1/4 cup almond flour

3 egg yolks

3 egg whites

1/4 cup coconut oil

1/4 cup nutmilk

1 teaspoon apple cider vinegar

1 teaspoon baking soda

1 teaspoon sea salt

Filling

8 oz ground meat (beef, chicken, turkey, etc.)

1 teaspoon ground black pepper

1 teaspoon paprika

1/2 teaspoon sea salt

1/2 small onion

1 mini dill pickle (or 1/2 large dill pickle)

Organic mustard

INSTRUCTIONS

1. Preheat oven to 325 degrees F. Line sheet pan with parchment paper or coat with coconut oil.
2. Preheat oven.
3. Place cashews, egg yolks, nut milk, coconut oil and vinegar in a food processor or bullet blender. Process until smooth. Add coconut flour, almond flour and salt. Process again until a smooth, wet dough forms.
4. Beat egg whites in medium bowl with hand mixer until stiff peaks form. Add wet dough to egg whites with and blend until combined.
5. Wet hands and shape dough into 12 mini buns, similar to burger patties. Wet hands in between each bun.
6. Place buns on prepared sheet pan and bake for 10 -15 minutes, until golden and cooked through.
7. Heat large skillet or griddle over medium-high heat.
8. Mix ground meat with spices. Form into 12 mini patties. Place burgers on hot skillet or griddle and cook about 5 minutes, or until medium-well. Flip half way through cooking.
9. Remove buns from oven and allow to cool about 5 minutes.
10. Slices bun in half. Thinly slice onion and pickle. Place hamburger on bottom half of bun. Top with onion and pickle. Add mustard to taste. Top with top bun.
11. Serve warm.

Quick Chili

Prep Time: 5 minutes

Cook Time: 20 minutes

Servings: 4

INGREDIENTS

1 lb lean grass-fed ground beef (or elk, bison, turkey or chicken)

15 oz (1 can) organic tomato sauce

6 oz (1 can) organic tomato paste

1 small onion

1 bell pepper

2 cloves garlic

2 tablespoons chili powder

1 tablespoon ground cumin

1 tablespoon smoked paprika (or paprika)

1 teaspoon Mexican oregano (or dried oregano)

1 teaspoon ground black pepper

1 teaspoon sea salt

1/2 teaspoon cayenne pepper

1 tablespoon coconut oil

sea salt, to taste

INSTRUCTIONS

1. Heat medium pot over medium-high heat. Add 1 tablespoon coconut oil.

2. Peel onion and garlic. Stem and seed bell pepper. Chop and add to food processor or bullet blender. Pulse until finely minced.

3. Add to skillet and sauté for about 1 minute. Add ground beef and spices. Brown beef for about 5 minutes. Stir with whisk to break up meat well, or wooden spoon to keep beef chunkier.

4. Add whole cans of tomato sauce and paste. Stir to combine.

5. Bring to a simmer, then reduce heat to medium and cover loosely with lid to prevent splatter. Simmer about 10 minutes. Stir occasionally.

6. Use large serving spoon or ladle to serve hot.

Simple Gazpacho + Tortilla Chips

Prep Time: 20 minutes

Cook Time: 10 minutes

Servings: 4

INGREDIENTS

Grain-Free Tortillas

Gazpacho

2 (11.5 oz) cans organic tomato juice (or 3 cups juiced tomatoes)

4 plum tomatoes

2 red bell peppers

1 red onion

1 cucumber

3 garlic cloves

1/4 cup apple cider vinegar

1/4 cup coconut oil (or 2 tablespoons coconut oil and 2 tablespoons flavorful oil [walnut, almond, sesame, etc.])

1 teaspoon cracked black pepper (or ground black pepper)

1/2 tablespoon sea salt

INSTRUCTIONS

1. Seed cucumber and tomatoes. Seed, stem and vein bell peppers. Peel onion and garlic. Dice veggies, mince garlic, and add to medium serving bowl.

2. Add tomato juice, vinegar, oil, salt and pepper, and mix well. Place in refrigerator.

3. Heat medium pan over medium-high heat and coat with coconut oil.

4. For *Tortilla Chips*, prepare *Grain-Free Tortillas*.

5. Add more coconut oil to hot pan and allow to heat up. Cut tortillas into wedges with pizza cutter or sharp knife.

6. Add tortilla wedges back to hot pan in single layer and cook about 30 seconds on each side, until golden and crisp. Drain on paper towel. Repeat with remaining tortilla wedges.

7. Transfer warm *Tortilla Chips* to serving dish. Serve immediately with chilled *Gazpacho*.

Sweet Potato Fries + Ketchup

Prep Time: 5 minutes

Cook Time: 35 minutes

Servings: 2

INGREDIENTS

Sweet Potato Fries

1 large sweet potato

2 tablespoons coconut oil

1/2 teaspoon ground black pepper

1/2 teaspoon ground paprika

1/2 teaspoon sea salt

1/4 teaspoon cayenne pepper (optional)

Ketchup

4 oz (1/2 can) organic tomato sauce

6 oz (1 can) organic tomato paste

1 tablespoon apple cider vinegar

1/2 teaspoon garlic powder

1/2 teaspoon onion powder

1/2 teaspoon ground black pepper

INSTRUCTIONS

1. Preheat oven to 450 degrees F. Line sheet pan with parchment or coat lightly with coconut oil.

2. Peel sweet potato if preferred, but do not rinse. Slice sweet potato into 1/4 inch strips and add to medium mixing bowl with coconut oil, black pepper, paprika and cayenne (optional). Toss potatoes until well coated.

3. Spread fries in well-spaced, single layer on sheet pan. Sprinkle salt over potatoes.

4. Place sheet pan in oven and bake for 10 minutes.

5. Carefully remove sheet pan and turn fries over with tongs or spatula. Place sheet pan bake into oven. Bake for another 10 minutes, or until golden and crispy.

6. While *Sweet Potato Fries* bake, add tomato sauce, tomato paste, vinegar, garlic powder, onion powder and black pepper to small pot.

7. Heat pot over medium heat and reduced for about 5 minutes, stirring occasionally.

8. Once reduced, remove pot from heat. Transfer ketchup to serving dish and refrigerate about 20 minutes.

9. Remove sheet pan from oven and serve *Sweet Potato Fries* hot with *Ketchup*.

Sausage And Peppers Sub

Prep Time: 20 minutes

Cook Time: 20 minutes

Servings: 4

INSTRUCTIONS

Long Rolls

4 Italian sausage links (pork, chicken, etc.)

1 yellow onion

1 green bell pepper

DIRECTIONS

1. Preheat oven to 350 degrees F. Line sheet pan with parchment paper, or lightly coat with coconut oil. Or lightly coat 6 mini loaf pans with coconut oil.
2. Prepare *Long Rolls* and place in oven.
3. Heat medium skillet over medium heat.
4. Add sausage to hot skillet and sear about 8 minutes.
5. Peel onion, and stem and seed bell pepper. Slice onion and pepper and add to skillet. Stir and sauté veggies.
6. Cooked sausage and veggies about 8 minutes, until sausage is cooked through and veggies are tender and caramelized.
7. Remove *Long Rolls* from oven and let cool about 2 minutes.
8. Slice rolls along side or split through top. Place cooked sausage on roll and top with peppers and onions.

9. Serve hot.

Tuna Sandwich

Prep Time: 10 minutes

Cook Time: 15 minutes

Servings: 1

INSTRUCTIONS

andwich Bread

7 oz (1 can) chunk light tuna

1/2 avocado

1/2 small red onion

1 small carrot

1 small celery stalk

1/2 small cucumber

1/2 lemon

1/2 teaspoon paprika

1/4 teaspoon cracked black pepper (or ground black pepper)

1/4 teaspoon sea salt

DIRECTIONS

1. Preheat oven to 350 degrees F. Lightly coat 6 mini round cake pans or medium loaf pan with coconut oil. Bring medium pot of lightly salted water to a boil.

2. Prepare *Sandwich Bread* and place in oven.

3. While bread bakes, drain tuna and add to small mixing bowl. Cut celery stalk and carrot in half length-wise. Peel onion and cucumber. Finely dice celery, carrot and onion. Add to bowl.

4. Slice avocado in half and scoop flesh of non-pit half into bowl. Preserve pitted half in airtight container with pit intact for freshness.

5. Add salt, pepper paprika and squeeze of 1/2 lemon into bowl. Mash together with fork until combined and smooth. Slice cucumber into 1/4 inch rounds.

6. Refrigerate tuna mixture if preferred.

7. Remove *Sandwich Bread* from oven and let cool about 5 minutes.

8. Slice bread and fill with tuna mixture. Top with cucumber slices.

9. Serve immediately.

Kelp Noodle Stir-Fry

Prep Time: 10 minutes

Cook Time: 10 minutes

Servings: 2

INSTRUCTIONS

1 (12 oz) package kelp noodles

8 oz grass-fed beef

1/2 sweet onion

1 red bell pepper

1 hot chili pepper

2 cloves garlic

1 inch piece fresh ginger

1/2 teaspoon paprika

1/2 teaspoon ground black pepper

1/4 teaspoon sea salt

Small bunch fresh cilantro

1 lime

Coconut oil (for cooking)

DIRECTIONS

1. Heat large skillet or medium cast-iron wok over high heat. Drain and rinse kelp noodles. Add to medium bowl and soak for 5 minutes in water and juice of 1/2 lime.

2. Stem and seed peppers. Peel onion, garlic and ginger. Dice beef into strips and add to medium mixing bowl. Mince chili pepper,

garlic and ginger. Add to beef with salt, pepper, paprika and 1 teaspoon coconut oil. Mix with wooden spoon to evenly coat beef.

3. Slice onion and bell pepper and add to hot skillet. Sauté about 2 minutes. Add seasoned beef to skillet and sauté another 2 minutes to brown.

4. Drain kelp noodles and add to skillet. Stir until beef is browned and cooked to about medium-well, kelp noodles are heated through, and veggies caramelize.

5. Remove skillet from heat and plate stir-fry. Chop fresh cilantro.

6. Top stir-fry with cilantro and squeeze of 1/2 lime.

7. Serve hot.

Shrimp Taco

Prep Time: 15 minutes

Cook Time: 20 minutes

Servings: 4

INGREDIENTS

Grain-Free Tortillas

Filling

12 oz medium shrimp

1/2 small red onion

1 fresh jalapeño or (2 oz pickled jalapeño)

1 garlic clove

1/2 inch piece ginger root

1/4 head cabbage (1 cup shredded)

Large bunch cilantro

1 avocado

1 tomato

2 limes

Coconut oil (for cooking)

INSTRUCTIONS

1. Heat large pan over medium-high heat and lightly coat with coconut oil.
2. Prepare *Grain-Free Tortillas*, with 4 smaller portions.

3. Keep tortillas warm and moist in oven set to WARM under damp paper towel.

4. Use clean paper towel to carefully wipe out pan. Add 1 tablespoon coconut oil to pan.

5. Peel and devein shrimp, and remove tail. Peel and mince garlic and ginger. Peel and thinly slice onion. Slice fresh jalapeños.

6. Add shrimp to pan with garlic, ginger, onion and jalapeños. Sauté about 2 minutes, then squeeze juice of 1 lime and sprinkle pinch of salt and pepper over shrimp.

7. Sauté shrimp until just cooked, about 5 minutes. Remove from heat.

8. Grate radish, shred cabbage, dice tomato. Slice avocado in half, remove pit, and slice flesh in peel. Chop cilantro.

9. Remove tortillas from oven and layer with sautéed shrimp and onions. Top with shredded cabbage, radish, tomato and avocado slices. Finish with large pinch of cilantro and squeeze of lime.

10. Fold tortillas and serve warm.

Spicy Mango Fried Rice

Prep Time: 10 minutes

Cook Time: 15 minutes

Servings: 4

INGREDIENTS

1 head cauliflower

8 oz boneless, skinless chicken

1 mango

1 hot chili pepper

2 scallions

2 garlic cloves

3 tablespoons pure fish sauce (or coconut aminos)

3 teaspoons sesame oil (or walnut or almond oil)

1/2 teaspoon red pepper flake

1/2 lime

Coconut oil (for cooking)

INSTRUCTIONS

1. Heat large skillet or medium cast-iron wok over high heat. Lightly coat with coconut oil.
2. Cut cauliflower into florets and add to food processor with shredding attachment to rice. Or finely mince cauliflower.
3. Peel garlic and ginger and mince. Mince chili pepper. Thinly slice scallions. Carefully peel and dice mango. Dice chicken.

4. Add diced chicken, garlic, ginger, chili pepper and red pepper flake to hot skillet or wok. Sauté until chicken is golden brown and just cooked, about 3 minutes. Remove chicken and set aside.
5. Add cauliflower to hot pan or wok. Sauté about 5 minutes, until cauliflower is golden and a bit softened.
6. Add mango and scallions and cook another 2 - 5minutes, until cauliflower is cooked through.
7. Add chicken to cauliflower and stir.
8. Remove from heat and serve hot with a squeeze of lime.

Seared Tuna Salad

Prep Time: 10 minutes

Cook Time: 10 minutes

Servings: 1

INGREDIENTS

1 cup spinach

1 cup arugula

1 avocado

Seared Tuna

6 oz sushi-grade tuna steak

1 tablespoon sesame oil (or coconut oil)

Juice of 1/2 lemon

1 glove garlic

1/2 inch piece fresh ginger

1 teaspoon sesame seeds

Ginger Glaze

1/2 cup pure fish sauce (or coconut aminos)

1/4 cup apple cider vinegar

Juice of 1 1/2 lemons

2 tablespoons sweetener*

1 inch piece fresh ginger

1 green onion

INSTRUCTIONS

1. For *Ginger Glaze*, peel and grate fresh ginger and slice scallion. Add to small pot with fish sauce, vinegar, sweetener and lemon juice. Heat over medium heat and bring to a simmer. Simmer 5 - 7 minutes, until slightly reduced and thickened. Stir occasionally. Once reduced, transfer to serving dish and refrigerate.

2. For *Seared Tuna*, peel and grate or mince ginger and garlic. Add to small dish with lemon juice and sesame oil and mix to combine. Roll tuna steak in marinade to coat and let sit in dish for 10 minutes in refrigerator.

3. Slice avocado in half and pit. Slice flesh in peel. Place halves together to keep avocado from browning while continuing.

4. Heat small skillet over medium-high heat. Add 1 tablespoon coconut oil.

5. Place marinated tuna in hot oiled pan and sear on each side about 1 minute, until outer flesh is just crisped but inside *is not* cooked through. About 5 minutes.

6. Remove tuna and sprinkle with sesame seeds. Cut tuna into slices.

7. Plate spinach and arugula. Fan out avocado slices over salad.

8. Top salad with *Seared Tuna*. Drizzle on chilled *Ginger Glaze* and serve immediately.

*stevia, raw honey or agave nectar

Delectable Dinner Ideas

Parchment Baked Salmon

Prep Time: 5 minutes

Cook Time: 20 minutes

Servings: 1

INGREDIENTS

8 oz salmon fillet (deboned, skin-on)

6 - 8 medium asparagus stalks

1/2 lemon

1 basil sprig

1 rosemary sprig

1 teaspoon coconut oil

Pinch black pepper

Pinch sea salt

Parchment paper

Kitchen twine

INSTRUCTIONS

1. Place large sheet pan on bottom rack of oven. Preheat oven to 400 degrees F. prepare parchment sheet.

2. Place salmon in middle of parchment sheet skin-side down and sprinkle with salt and pepper. Place asparagus stalks next to salmon. Cut lemon into thin slices and place over fish and asparagus. Rub herbs between palms, then lay basil and rosemary sprig over lemon slices. Drizzle 1 teaspoon coconut oil over salmon and asparagus.

3. Gather edges of parchment up over salmon and tie tightly with kitchen twine to form sealed pouch.
4. Place pouch directly on hot baking sheet in hot oven. Bake for 20 minutes.
5. Remove from oven and carefully transfer pouch to serving plate. Carefully open pouch to release steam.
6. Serve hot.

Smoked Salmon Eggs Benedict

Prep Time: 15 minutes

Cook Time: 25 minutes

Servings: 4

INGREDIENTS

4 cage free eggs

6 oz smoked salmon

2 sprigs fresh dill

English Muffins

1/3 cup coconut flour

1/3 cup almond flour

2 eggs

1/4 cup almond milk (or low-fat coconut milk)

2 tablespoons coconut oil

1/2 teaspoon baking soda

1 teaspoon apple cider vinegar

Hollandaise Sauce

1/2 cup ghee or coconut oil (melted)

2 egg yolks

1/2 lemon

1/4 teaspoon sea salt

INSTRUCTIONS

1. Preheat oven to 400 degrees F. Coat 2 mini-round cake pans or 4-inch diameter ceramic ramekins with coconut oil. Bring medium pot to simmer with 1 teaspoon salt and 1 teaspoon apple cider vinegar.

2. For *English Muffins*, mix baking soda and apple cider vinegar In small bowl. Set aside and allow to froth.

3. In medium mixing bowl, beat egg whites with hand mixer or whisk until thick and frothy. Add yolks, almond and coconut flour, nut milk, and coconut oil. Mix gently.

4. Add baking soda and vinegar mixture to bowl and blend well until smooth and free of clumps.

5. Pour batter into pans or ramekins and place on sheet pan. Place in oven and bake 15 -18 minutes, until golden brown and center is firm to the touch.

6. Crack eggs into 4 separate small bowls. Coat or spray metal ladle with coconut oil. Hold ladle over simmering water and pour 1 egg into coated ladle. Slowly tilt edge of ladle into hot water, filling it gently while keeping ladle just submerged in water. Do not let egg float out of ladle or submerge ladle into water entirely. Hold and cook egg about 1 - 2 minutes, until whites are opaque and yolk is warmed but still runny. Place poached egg on paper towel to drain. Repeat with remaining eggs.

7. Remove muffins from oven. Loosen from sides of cake pans or ramekins with knife and turn out onto wire rack to cool.

8. For *Hollandaise Sauce*, add egg yolks, squeeze of lemon, and salt to food processor or high-speed blender. Processor for 30 seconds. While processor or blender is running, drizzle in melted ghee or coconut oil very slowly. Process until all fat is added and emulsified and sauce thickens a bit, about 2 minutes.

9. Cut slightly cool *English Muffins* in half and transfer to serving dish.

10. Layer *English Muffin* halves with smoked salmon, then top with a poached egg. Pour *Hollandaise Sauce* over poached eggs, to taste. Sprinkle with pinch of salt and cracked black pepper, if preferred. Chop dill and sprinkle over eggs.

11. Serve immediately.

Steak Tartar with Truffle Tapenade

Prep Time: 15 minutes

Servings: 2

INGREDIENTS

Steak Tartar

8 oz beef tenderloin

1 anchovy fillet

1 egg yolk (optional)

1 tablespoon organic mustard

2 tablespoons coconut oil

1 garlic clove

1 shallot

1/2 teaspoon ground black pepper

1/4 teaspoon sea salt

Small bunch fresh parsley

Truffle Tapenade

1 cup pitted olives (Kalamata, Spanish or other gourmet variety)

2 teaspoons capers

1 small black truffle

1 small lemon

2 tablespoons truffle oil (or coconut oil)

1/4 teaspoon sea salt

Small bunch basil leaves

INSTRUCTIONS

1. For *Steak Tartar*, peel and crush garlic and shallot with pestle in medium mixing bowl. Or mince and add to bowl with anchovy, mustard, egg yolk, salt and pepper.

2. Whisk in coconut oil to form emulsion. Finely dice tenderloin and add to bowl. Toss to combine and transfer to chilled serving dish.

3. For *Truffle Tapenade*, rinse and drain olives and capers. Place in food processor or high-speed blender with truffle oil and salt.

4. Squeeze lemon juice and shave about 1 1/2 tablespoons worth of black truffle into processor. Pulse until mixture is finely chopped but not smooth. Transfer to serving dish with *Steak Tartar*.

5. Finely chop parsley and garnish *Steak Tartar*. Finely chop or chiffon basil and garnish *Truffle Tapenade*.

6. Serve immediately. Or refrigerate 20 minutes and serve chilled.

Kelp Noodle Salad with Crunchy Cashew Sauce

Prep Time: 10 minutes*

Servings: 2

INGREDIENTS

1 package (12 oz) kelp noodles

1/2 lemon

1 small red bell pepper

1 small carrot

Small bunch basil leaves

Crunchy Cashew Sauce

1 cup raw cashews

1 orange

1/2 lemon

1/2 teaspoon paprika

1/2 teaspoon ground oregano

1/2 teaspoon ground black pepper

1/2 teaspoon sea salt

INSTRUCTIONS

1. *Soak 3/4 cup cashews in enough water to cover at least 4 hours. Drain and rinse.

2. Rinse and drain kelp noodles. Add to medium bowl and soak 5 minutes in warm water and juice of 1/2 lemon.

3. Cut bell pepper in half, then remove stem, seeds and veins. Thinly slice bell pepper lengthwise. Use vegetable peeler or grater to make long, thin slices of carrot. Add veggies to medium mixing bowl.

4. For *Crunchy Cashew Sauce*, add soaked cashews, juice of lemon and orange, salt and spices to food processor or bullet. Process until very smooth.

5. Add drained kelp noodles to mixing bowl. Pour *Crunchy cashew Sauce* over veggies and kelp noodles. Chiffon basil leaves and chop remaining unsoaked cashews. Sprinkle over bowl.

6. Toss to coat. Transfer to serving dishes and serve immediately.

7. Or refrigerate for 20 minutes and serve chilled.

Quick Raw Avocado Slaw

Prep Time: 10 minutes*

Cook Time: 20 minutes

Servings: 4

INGREDIENTS

1/2 head cabbage (2 cups shredded)

1 avocado

1 carrot

Zest of 1 lemon

Juice of 1 lemon

1 tablespoon raw honey

2 tablespoons apple cider vinegar

1 teaspoon ground white pepper (or black pepper)

1 teaspoon sea salt

INSTRUCTIONS

1. Cut avocado in half and remove pit. Scoop flesh into large mixing bowl and mash with fork.
2. Remove any tough outer leaves and core from cabbage. Shred cabbage and carrot. Add to bowl with vinegar, honey, salt and pepper. Zest *then* juice lemon, and add.
3. Toss to combine.
4. Serve immediately. Or and place in refrigerator for 20 minutes and serve chilled.

Mango Ginger Apple Salad

Prep Time: 5 minutes

Servings: 2

INSTRUCTIONS

1 ripe mango

1 granny smith apple

1/4 cup raw cashews

1 inch piece fresh ginger

1/2 teaspoon ground ginger

INGREDIENTS

1. Slice mango in half around pit. Peel flesh and dice. Add to small mixing bowl.
2. Core apple and dice. Peel ginger and mince. Add to bowl with ground ginger.
3. Roughly chop cashews and add to bowl.
4. Mix well and serve immediately. Or refrigerate 20 minutes and serve chilled.

Chicken Fries with Garlic Aioli

Prep Time: 10 minutes

Cook Time: 15 minutes

Servings: 2

INGREDIENTS

8 oz boneless, skinless chicken breast

1 egg

1/2 cup almond meal

1 teaspoon flax meal (or ground chia seed)

1 teaspoon ground black pepper

1/2 teaspoon paprika

1/2 teaspoon onion powder

1/2 teaspoon garlic powder

1/2 teaspoon chili powder

1/2 teaspoon sea salt

Garlic Aioli

1/2 - 3/4 cup coconut oil

1 egg yolk

2 garlic cloves

1/2 small lemon

1/4 teaspoon ground white pepper (or black pepper)

1/4 teaspoon sea salt

3 tablespoons flavorful oil (black truffle, walnut, almond, sesame, etc.)
(optional)

INSTRUCTIONS

1. Heat large pan over medium-high heat and coat with coconut oil.

2. For *Garlic Aioli*, peel garlic and add to food processor or blender with egg yolk, juice of 1/2 lemon, salt and pepper. Process until smooth, scraping down sides of vessel.

3. While processor or blender is running, very slowly drizzle in enough coconut oil to create thick mayo-like mixture. Drizzle in flavorful oil as well will processor runs (optional). If mixture is runny, drizzle in more coconut oil while processor runs until thickened. Pour into serving dish and refrigerate.

4. Slice chicken into half width-wise, creating twice the fillets. Try to slice at thickest portion to keep all fillets equal thickness.

5. Slice chicken fillets into long, 1/2 inch wide strips. Place strips between two paper towels and press to absorb excess moisture.

6. In a shallow dish, blend almond meal, flax or chia meal, spices and salt.

7. Beat egg in small mixing bowl. Toss chicken strips in beaten egg to lightly coat, then dredge in seasoned almond meal.

8. Carefully place coated chicken strips into hot oil and fry about 2 - 3 minutes, until golden brown and cooked through. Turn with tongs half way through cooking.

9. Drain cooked chicken on paper towel, then transfer to serving dish.

10. Serve hot with *Garlic Aioli*.

Chicken Noodle Soup

Prep Time: 10 minutes

Cook Time: 20 minutes

Servings: 2

INGREDIENTS

Noodles

1/2 cup almond flour

1/2 cup arrowroot powder

1/2 cup tapioca flour

1 egg

2 egg yolks

1 tablespoon coconut oil

1/2 teaspoon sea salt

Soup

8 oz skin-on chicken

1 1/2 cup chicken broth or stock

1/2 cup water

2 carrots

1 celery stalk

2 teaspoons dried thyme (4 teaspoons fresh thyme)

1/2 teaspoon black pepper

Pinch sea salt

INSTRUCTIONS

1. Heat medium pot over medium-high heat. Place chicken skin-side down in hot pot. Sear and render out fat for about 5 minutes.

2. Dice carrots and celery. Add to chicken with salt and pepper.

3. Turn chicken and brown on flesh side about 5 minutes. Stir veggies as well.

4. Add thyme, chicken stock and water, and increase heat to high. Bring soup to simmer. Adjust heat as necessary and keep at simmer or soft boil.

5. For *Noodles*, sift almond flour, tapioca flour, 1/3 cup arrow powder and salt into medium mixing bowl. Make well in the center of flour mixture and add egg and yolks. Whisk eggs into flour in circular motion with a fork until dough pulls together.

6. Dust cutting board with half of remaining arrowroot powder. Turn dough out onto cutting board and knead for 5 minutes, until smooth.

7. Add 1 tablespoon coconut oil if dough is too dry. Add 1 tablespoon almond flour at a time if dough is too moist or sticky.

8. Dust cutting board with remaining arrowroot powder. Roll dough into rectangular shape with a rolling pin to about 1/8 inch thickness. Cut pasta sheet into long strips with pizza cutter or sharp knife. Or run past through pasta machine several times until desired thickness is reached. Then use cutting attachment to cut pasta into preferred style.

9. Separate noodles a bit and place gently in simmering soup for about 3 minutes.
10. Transfer to serving dish and serve immediately.

Cheese Steak Sandwich

Prep Time: 10 minutes*

Cook Time: 15 minutes

Servings: 4

INGREDIENTS

Long Roll

Almond Cheese

1 cup soaked skinless almonds*

1 tablespoons lemon juice

1 tablespoon apple cider vinegar

1 garlic clove

1/4 teaspoon ground black pepper

1/4 teaspoon paprika

1/2 teaspoon sea salt

1/4 cup water or 2 tablespoons coconut oil

Filling

1 lb beef steak

1 small onion

1 small bell pepper

1/2 teaspoon ground black pepper

1/2 teaspoon Sea salt

INSTRUCTIONS

1. *Soak almonds in enough water to cover overnight. Drain and rinse.

2. Preheat oven to 350 degrees F. Line sheet pan with parchment paper, or lightly coat with coconut oil. Or lightly coat 6 mini loaf pans with coconut oil.

3. Prepare *Long Rolls* and place in oven.

4. While bread bakes, heat medium skillet over medium-high heat.

5. Peel onion. Stem, vein and seed pepper. Thinly slice steak, onion and pepper.

6. Add steak to hot skillet and sauté about 1 minute. Add veggies, salt and pepper. Sauté about 5 minutes, until meat is cooked and veggies are soft and caramelized. Remove from heat.

7. Remove *Long Rolls* from oven and let cool about 2 minutes.

8. Add all *Almond Cheese* ingredients to food processor or bullet blender and process until smooth. Add 1 tablespoon water or coconut oil at a time to reach preferred consistency.

9. Slice roll along side or split through top and spread on *Almond Cheese*. Then layer on meat and veggies.

10. Serve immediately.

Mint Melon Salad

Prep Time: 15 minutes

Servings: 4

INGREDIENTS

1/4 watermelon (about 1 lb)

1/2 honeydew melon

1 small cucumber

2 fresh mint sprigs

1 fresh basil sprig

1/4 cup organic champagne (or sparkling wine or sparkling apple cider)

INSTRUCTIONS

1. Cut flesh from watermelon and honeydew rind, and peel cucumber and seed cucumber. Chop and add to medium mixing bowl.
2. Or use melon baller to remove flesh of melons and peeled cucumber, and add to medium mixing bowl.
3. Remove mint and basil leaves from stalks and chiffon or mince. Add to bowl with champagne. Set aside in refrigerator for 10 minutes.
4. Transfer to serving dish and serve chilled.

Shrimp Stuffed Squid

Prep Time: 15 minutes

Cook Time: 25 minutes

Servings: 4

INGREDIENTS

Stuffed Squid

12 medium whole squid (calamari)

8 oz medium shrimp

2 cups baby spinach

1/3 cup almond flour

1 egg

1 tablespoon apple cider vinegar

3 garlic cloves

Small bunch fresh oregano

1/4 teaspoon crushed red pepper flakes

3/4 teaspoon sea salt

2 tablespoons coconut oil

8 wooden toothpicks

Sauce

16 oz (2 cans) organic tomato sauce

1 small onion

2 garlic cloves

1/2 cup dry white wine (or 1/3 cup sparkling apple cider + 3 tablespoons apple cider vinegar)

INSTRUCTIONS

1. Have fishmonger clean squid and peel and devein shrimp. Or clean and rinse squid and peel and devein shrimp yourself.

2. Heat medium pan over medium heat. Add coconut oil to pan.

3. Peel garlic and add to food processor or high-speed blender with shrimp and 4 squid. Pulse until coarse paste forms.

4. Add shrimp paste to medium mixing bowl. Roughly chop spinach and oregano leaves and add to bowl with egg, almond flour, vinegar, red pepper and salt. Mix to combine.

5. Stuff remaining squid bodies with stuffing. Secure closed with toothpicks.

6. Use tongs to add stuffed and secured squid to hot oiled pan. Sear for about 1 minute, then flip.

7. Peel and roughly chop onion and garlic. Add to food processor or high-speed blender with white wine. Process until onion and garlic are well broken down.

8. Pour mixture over seared squid. Add tomato sauce and gently stir to blend. Cover and simmer squid in sauce for 15 minutes.

9. Turn over stuffed squid and continue cooking uncovered another 10 minutes.

10. Remove pan from heat. Remove squid from pan and remove toothpicks from squid with tongs or forks.

11. Transfer squid to serving dish and pour sauce over.

12. Serve hot.

Veggie Burger

Prep Time: 5 minutes

Cook Time: 20 minutes

Servings: 4

INGREDIENTS

Soft Burger Bun

Veggie Burger

2 eggs

1/2 head cauliflower

2 medium carrots

1 small white onion

1 cup walnuts (1/2 cup ground)

1/4 cup almond flour

2 tablespoons tapioca flour

2 tablespoons ground chia seed (or flax meal)

2 cloves garlic

1 teaspoon paprika

1 teaspoon ground black pepper

1 teaspoon sea salt

Topping

1 avocado

1 heirloom tomato

1 white onion

2 ribs romaine lettuce (or preferred lettuce)

INSTRUCTIONS

1. Preheat oven to 350 degrees F. Line sheet pan with parchment paper, or lightly coat with coconut oil. Or lightly coat 6 mini round cake pans with coconut oil.
2. Prepare *Soft Burger Buns* and place in oven.
3. While bread bakes, line dish with parchment paper.
4. Add walnuts and almond four to food processor or bullet blender. Process until finely ground. Add to medium mixing bowl.
5. Peel small onion and garlic. Add to processor or blender with cauliflower and carrots. Process until finely ground. Add eggs, tapioca and chia. Process until mixture becomes thickened and has batter-like consistency.
6. Add veggie mixture and spices to mixing bowl. Mix all ingredients together with hands or wooden spoon until fully combined and uniform.
7. Form veggie mixture into 4 patties and place on parchment lined dish. Place in freezer for 10 minutes.
8. Heat medium skillet over medium-high heat and add 1 tablespoon coconut oil.
9. Peel onion. Make 4 thick slices, keeping full ring intact. Using spatula, place full rings into hot oiled pan. Sear 1 minute on each side. Set aside on paper towel to drain.
10. Reduce heat to medium and coat pan with coconut oil.

11. Remove veggie patties from freezer and place in hot oiled pan. Cook 5 minutes, then carefully flip with spatula and cook another 5 minutes.
12. Remove *Soft Burger Bun* from oven and let cool about 5 minutes.
13. Cut lettuce ribs in half. Cut tomato into 4 thick slices. Slice avocado in half, pit and slice flesh in peel.
14. Slice bun in half and place lettuce on bottom bun, followed by tomato slice. Add burger patty, then grilled onion ring. Finish with a few slices of avocado and top bun.
15. Serve immediately.

Crisp Spinach Salad

Prep Time: 15 minutes

Cook Time: 15 minutes

Servings: 2

INGREDIENTS

Spinach Salad

4 cups spinach

2 eggs

8 slices nitrate-free bacon

1 avocado

1 small onion

1/4 cup almond flour

1/2 teaspoon ground black pepper

1/4 teaspoon paprika

1/4 teaspoon sea salt

Bacon Vinaigrette

Bacon drippings

2 tablespoons coconut oil

2 tablespoons apple cider vinegar

1 teaspoon sweetener*

2 teaspoons organic mustard

1/4 teaspoon ground black pepper

INSTRUCTIONS

1. Bring small pot of lightly salted water to boil. Heat medium skillet over medium-high heat.

2. Gently add eggs to boiling water with tongs and boil about 7 - 10 minutes. Then remove and rinse under cold water. Crack shells and remove whole egg. Set aside.

3. While eggs cook, chop bacon and add to hot pan. Sauté about 5 - 8 minutes, until crisp and cooked through. Remove bacon and drain on paper towel. Reserve bacon drippings. Add drippings to small bowl once cooled slightly.

4. Lightly coat hot pan with coconut oil.

5. Add almond flour and spiced to small mixing bowl. Peel onion and cut in half. Cut onion into half-moon slices. Toss with almond flour until well coated.

6. Add coated onions to hot oiled pan. Let crisp about 1 - 2 minutes, then turn and continue cooking another minute, until fully crisp. Remove onion crisps and set aside on paper towel to drain.

7. Rinse, dry and plate spinach. Slice avocado in half, pit, and slice in peel. Slice eggs.

8. Add bacon pieces, avocado slices, sliced eggs and onion crisp to salads.

9. Add *Bacon Vinaigrette* ingredients to small bowl with reserved bacon grease and whisk well. Pour over salads.

10. Serve immediately.

*stevia raw honey or agave nectar

Chicken Pot Pie

Prep Time: 15 minutes

Cook Time: 30 minutes

Servings: 4

INGREDIENTS

Filling

8 oz skin-on chicken

1 1/2 cup chicken broth

2 tablespoons tapioca flour

2 tablespoons coconut oil

2 carrots

1 celery stalk

1 green bell pepper

1 small onion

2 garlic cloves

2 teaspoons dried thyme (or 4 teaspoons fresh thyme)

1 tablespoon lemon juice

1/2 teaspoon black pepper

Pinch sea salt

Crust

1/3 cup almond flour

2 tablespoons coconut flour

3 tablespoons cold coconut oil (or cacao butter)

1 egg

3 - 4 teaspoons water

1/2 teaspoon dried thyme

1/4 teaspoon sea salt

INSTRUCTIONS

1. Preheat oven to 400 degrees F. Heat medium pot over medium heat.

2. Add two tablespoon coconut oil to hot pot. Add chicken pieces skin side down. Cook about 3 minutes, then turn with tongs and continue cooking another 3 minutes. Remove chicken and set aside.

3. Whisk coconut flour into pot until smooth. Gradually whisk in chicken broth. Simmer about 5 minutes, whisking occasionally.

4. Peel and mince garlic. Chop carrots, celery, onion and bell pepper. Add to pot with thyme, salt pepper and lemon juice.

5. Chop par-cooked chicken meat. Add back to pot and simmer for 5 minutes. Remove from heat and set aside.

6. For *Crust*, add cold coconut oil to flours, thyme and salt in small bowl. Cut fat into flour with fork until crumbly. Mix in egg and enough water to bring together tender dough.

7. Divide dough into 4 portions. Roll into balls and flatten into round disks large enough to fit over mini pie tins or ceramic ramekins with hand, then rolling pin.

8. Pour *Filling* into vessels and cover with crusts. Pinch edges of dough over edges of vessels to seal in liquid. Brush top of each pie with coconut oil, coconut milk, or egg wash and sprinkle with salt. Use knife to cut a slit in the top of each pie.

9. Bake pot pies for about 15 minutes, until crust is golden.

10. Remove from oven and allow pies to cool for 10 minutes.

11. Serve warm. Or let cool completely and serve room temperature.

Lamb Pot Pie

Prep Time: 15 minutes

Cook Time: 30 minutes

Servings: 4

INGREDIENTS

Filling

8 oz lamb

1 1/2 cup beef or vegetable broth

2 tablespoons tapioca flour

2 tablespoons coconut oil

2 chopped carrots

1 chopped celery stalk

1 bell pepper (yellow, orange or red)

1 small green tomato (or under ripe red tomato)

1 small onion

2 garlic cloves

1 inch piece ginger

1 tablespoon curry powder

1 tablespoon ground coriander

1 teaspoon ground cumin

1/2 teaspoon ground cinnamon

1/2 teaspoon black pepper

Pinch sea salt

Crust

1/3 cup almond flour

2 tablespoons coconut flour

3 tablespoons cold coconut oil (or cacao butter)

1 egg

3 - 4 teaspoons water

1/2 teaspoon turmeric

1/4 teaspoon sea salt

INSTRUCTIONS

1. Preheat oven to 400 degrees F. Heat medium pot over medium heat.

2. Add two tablespoon coconut oil to hot pot. Add lamb. Sauté about 5 minutes, then remove lamb with tongs.

3. Whisk in coconut flour until smooth. Gradually whisk in broth. Simmer about 5 minutes, whisking occasionally.

4. Peel and mince garlic and ginger. Chop carrots, celery, onion, bell pepper and tomato. Add to pot with salt, and spices.

5. Chop par-cooked lamb meat. Add lamb back to pot and simmer for 5 minutes. Remove from heat and set aside.

6. For *Crust*, add cold coconut oil to flours, turmeric and salt in small bowl. Cut fat into flour with fork until crumbly. Mix in egg and enough water to bring together tender dough.

7. Divide dough into 4 portions. Roll into balls and flatten into round disks large enough to fit over mini pie tins or ceramic ramekins with hand, then rolling pin.

8. Pour *Filling* into vessels and cover with crusts. Pinch edges of dough over edges of vessels to seal in liquid. Brush top of each pie with coconut oil, coconut milk, or egg wash and sprinkle with salt. Use knife to cut a slit in the top of each pie.
9. Bake pot pies for about 15 minutes, until crust is golden.
10. Remove from oven and allow pies to cool for 10 minutes.
11. Serve warm. Or let cool completely and serve room temperature.

Meatballs

Prep Time: 5 minutes

Cook Time: 20 minutes

Servings: 4

INGREDIENTS

16 oz (1 lb) ground meat (beef, pork, chicken, bison, or any combination)

1 cup almond flour

1 egg

1 garlic clove

1/2 small onion

1 teaspoon dried parsley

1 teaspoon dried oregano

1/2 teaspoon ground black pepper

1/2 teaspoon sea salt

Tomato Sauce

4 oz organic tomato sauce

4 oz organic crushed tomatoes

1 teaspoon dried oregano

1/2 teaspoon dried basil

1/2 teaspoon ground black pepper

DIRECTIONS

1. Preheat oven to 350 degrees. Line baking sheet with parchment or baking mat. Or prepare glass or ceramic casserole dish.

2. Pulse onion and garlic in food processor or blender until finely processed, but before paste forms. Or finely mince onion and garlic.

3. Beat egg in large bowl. Add ground meat, almond flour, spices and salt. Mix well with hands or large wooden spoon.

4. Form 18 - 24 meatballs with scoop or tablespoon, then roll in hands.

5. Arrange meatballs on lines sheet pan or in casserole dish and bake for 15 to 20 minutes, until golden brown and cooked through.

6. Add all *Tomato Sauce* ingredients to small pot and heat over medium heat. Stir and simmer about 10 minutes, until reduced and thickened.

7. Remove meatballs from oven. Toss with *Tomato Sauce* and serve hot.

8. Or allow meatballs and *Tomato Sauce* to cool, then pack in lidded containers. Serve room temperature.

Jamaican Jerk Patty

Prep Time: 20 minutes

Cook Time: 30 minutes

Servings: 4

INSTRUCTIONS

Crust

2 cups almond flour

2 eggs

3 tablespoons coconut oil

1 teaspoon curry powder

1/4 teaspoon baking soda

1/2 teaspoon sea salt

Filling

8 oz meat (ground or shredded chicken, beef or pork)

1 small onion

1 tablespoon curry powder

1 teaspoon allspice

1 teaspoon chile powder

1 teaspoon cayenne pepper

1 teaspoon red pepper flake

1/2 teaspoon garlic powder

1/2 teaspoon onion powder

1/2 teaspoon ground cinnamon

DIRECTIONS

1. For *Crust*, sift almond flour into medium mixing bowl. Add baking soda, curry powder and salt.

2. Whisk eggs in small mixing bowl, then add to flour and combine. Slowly add coconut oil until malleable dough comes together.

3. Roll in plastic wrap or wrap tightly in parchment and refrigerate for 15 minutes.

4. Preheat oven to 400 degrees. Line sheet pan with parchment or baking mat. Cover cutting board with parchment. Heat medium pan over medium heat.

5. Peel and mince onion. Add to hot pan with ground or shredded meat and spices. Sauté about 5 - 10 minutes, until beef is browned. Remove from heat and set aside.

6. Remove dough from refrigerator. Divide dough into 4 portions. Roll dough into balls and flatten on parchment covered cutting board with hands. Roll into circles about 1/8 inch thick with rolling pin.

7. Scoop equal portions of *Filling* into center of one side of dough circle. Fold bare half of dough over filled half. Press edges together, letting any trapped air escape. Crimp edges of dough together with fork. Repeat with remaining dough.

8. Arrange patties on lined sheet pan and bake 15 - 20 minutes, or until dough is golden and cooked through.

9. Serve immediately. Or allow to cool and store in air-tight container.

Chicken Tenders

Prep Time: 5 minutes

Cook Time: 10 minutes

Servings: 2

INGREDIENTS

8 oz boneless, skinless chicken

1 egg

1/2 cup almond meal

1 teaspoon flax meal

1 teaspoon paprika

1/2 teaspoon thyme

1/2 teaspoon onion powder

1/2 teaspoon ground black pepper

1/2 teaspoon sea salt

Honey Mustard

2 tablespoon raw honey or agave nectar

3 tablespoons organic mustard

INSTRUCTIONS

1. Heat a medium skillet over medium high heat. Lightly coat pan with coconut oil.
2. Slice chicken into 1 inch wide strips. Arrange slices between 2 sheets of parchment and pound with kitchen mallet or rolling

pin to flatten slightly. Place flattened pieces between two paper towels to absorb excess moisture.

3. In a shallow dish, blend almond meal, flax meal, spices and salt.

4. Beat egg in small mixing bowl. Dip chicken into beaten egg, then dredge in seasoned almond meal.

5. Carefully place coated chicken strips into hot oil and fry about 3 - 4minutes, until golden brown and cooked through. Turn with tongs half way through cooking.

6. Drain cooked chicken on paper towel, then transfer to serving dish. Serve warm.

7. Or allow to cool and transfer to lidded container. Serve room temperature or chilled.

8. Mix mustard and sweetener in small serving bowl or lidded container. Serve with chicken.

*stevia, raw honey or agave nectar

Pizza Bites

Prep Time: 20 minutes*

Cook Time: 20 minutes

Servings: 4

INSTRUCTIONS

Crust

2 cups almond flour

2 eggs

3 tablespoons coconut oil

1/4 teaspoon baking soda

1 teaspoon sea salt

Almond Cheese

1 cup skinless almonds*

1/4 cup water

2 tablespoons coconut oil

1 tablespoon lemon juice

1 tablespoon apple cider vinegar

1 garlic clove

1/2 teaspoon sea salt

1/4 teaspoon ground white pepper (or black pepper)

Pizza Sauce

4 oz organic tomato paste

4 oz organic tomato sauce

1 teaspoon dried oregano

1/2 teaspoon dried basil

1/2 teaspoon ground black pepper

Filling

4 oz natural pepperoni

4 oz natural ground sausage

1/2 bell pepper

DIRECTIONS

1. *For *Almond Cheese*, soak almonds in 1 1/2 cups water overnight. Drain and rinse.

2. For *Crust*, sift almond flour into medium mixing bowl. Add baking soda, spices and salt.

3. Whisk eggs in small mixing bowl, then add to flour and combine. Slowly add coconut oil until malleable dough comes together.

4. Roll in plastic wrap or wrap tightly in parchment and refrigerate for 15 minutes.

5. Preheat oven to 400 degrees. Line sheet pan with parchment or baking mat. Cover cutting board with parchment. Heat medium pan over medium heat.

6. Seed and stem bell pepper. Dice pepper and pepperoni. Add peppers and sausage to hot pan. Sauté about 5 minutes, until sausage is cooked through. Transfer to small bowl to cool, and add diced pepperoni. Set aside.

7. Add all *Almond Cheese* ingredients to food processor or bullet blender and process until smooth. Add a few extra tablespoons of water if necessary to achieve thick but smooth consistency. Set aside.

8. In small bowl, mix together all *Pizza Sauce* ingredients. Set aside.

9. Remove dough from refrigerator. Roll dough out on parchment covered cutting board with rolling pin to about 1/8 inch thickness. Use sharp knife or pizza cutter to cut dough into 2x4 inch rectangles.

10. Spread *Almond Cheese* in center of one half of each dough piece. Then dollop with small amount of *Pizza Sauce*, and a pinch of *Filling*.

11. Fold over bare half of dough. Press edges together, pressing out any trapped air. Use fork to crimp edges for better seal. Repeat with remaining dough.

12. Arrange *Pizza Bites* on lined sheet pan and bake 15 - 20 minutes, or until dough is golden and cooked through.

13. Serve immediately. Or allow to cool and store in air-tight container.

Peppercorn Crusted Filet Mignon

Prep Time: 5 minutes

Cook Time: 5 minutes

Servings: 2

INGREDIENTS

2 (6 oz) filet mignon steaks

1 tablespoons ghee (or coconut oil)

1 tablespoon black peppercorns

1/2 teaspoon sea salt

1 tablespoons coconut oil

INSTRUCTIONS

1. Heat medium pan over medium-high heat and add 1 tablespoon coconut oil.

2. Place peppercorns in a plastic kitchen bag or parchment pouch and place on cutting board other counter. Crack peppercorns with heavy rolling pin or pan until broken.

3. Add cracked peppercorns to small mixing bowl with ghee or coconut oil and mix to combine.

4. Sprinkle steaks with salt , then rub with peppercorn mixture, coating evenly on both sides.

5. Place seasoned steaks in hot oiled pan and cook 2 - 4 minutes per side, for rare to medium rare. Carefully flip half way through cooking, and disturb only this once.

6. Transfer seared steaks a cutting board and let rest at least 5 minutes.
7. Serve warm with your favorite grilled veggies. Or slice with sharp knife and serve.

Orange Glazed Duck Breast

Prep Time: 5 minutes

Cook Time: 5 minutes

Servings: 2

INGREDIENTS

2 (8 oz) boneless duck breast halves

2 teaspoons dried thyme

1 sprig rosemary

1/2 teaspoon ground black pepper

1 teaspoons sea salt

2 tablespoons coconut oil (or bacon fat or ghee)

Orange Glaze

2 - 3 oranges

1/3 cup organic champagne (or sparkling apple cider)

1 teaspoon black peppercorns

1/2 inch piece fresh ginger

INSTRUCTIONS

1. Heat medium pan over medium-high heat. Add 2 tablespoons preferred fat to hot pan.

2. For *Orange Glaze*, zest 1 orange and add to small pan. Juice oranges and add to pan. Heat pan over high heat. Add champagne and peppercorns. Peel ginger and mince. Add to pan and stir. Bring to simmer, then reduce heat to medium.

Simmer until reduced by half, about 5 minutes. Then reduce heat to low. When desired thickness is reach, remove from heat and strain *Orange Glaze* into serving dish.

3. While *Orange Glaze* reduces, rinse duck breast and pat dry with paper towel. Rub rosemary spring between palms, then remove needles from stem. Roughly chop.

4. Rub rosemary, thyme, salt and pepper into both sides of duck breasts.

5. Place duck breasts in hot oiled pan, skin and fat side down. Let brown undisturbed for 5 minutes. Turn duck over with tongs and cook until desired doneness, 5 - 10 minutes for medium to well done.

6. Transfer duck breasts to cutting board and cover with aluminum foil. Set aside to rest 5 minutes.

7. Cut each duck breast in 1/2 inch diagonally slices. Arrange sliced duck breasts on plates and drizzle on desired amount of *Orange Glaze*.

8. Serve sliced duck breasts warm with side of *Orange Glaze*.

Clams Casino

Prep Time: 5 minutes

Cook Time: 25 minutes

Servings: 4

INGREDIENTS

18 medium littleneck clams

1/3 cup dry white wine (or 1/4 cup sparkling apple cider + 2 tablespoons apple cider vinegar)

4 - 6 slices nitrate-free bacon

1 large red bell pepper

4 shallots

2 large garlic cloves

1/3 cup almonds

1/4 teaspoon dried oregano

1/4 teaspoon ground black pepper

1/4 teaspoon sea salt

2 tablespoons coconut oil

INSTRUCTIONS

1. Have fishmonger shuck clams and loosen meat from bottom shell. Reserve bottom shell.

2. Heat large pan over medium-high heat and add coconut oil. Line sheet pan with parchment or aluminum foil.

3. Finely chop bacon and add to hot pan. Sauté until crisp, about 5 minutes. Use slotted spoon to remove cooked bacon from pan and drain on paper towel. Set aside.

4. Preheat oven to 500 degrees F.

5. Remove seeds, stem and veins from bell pepper, then finely chop. Peel and finely chop shallots. Peel and mince garlic. Add to hot bacon drippings with oregano, salt and pepper. Sauté about 5 minutes, until shallots are tender and translucent.

6. Add wine to pan and simmer until just evaporated, about 2 minutes. Remove pan from heat and stir in reserved bacon.

7. Arrange clams in bottom shells on prepared sheet pan. Spoon bacon mixture onto the clams, packing slightly into mound.

8. Finely chop almonds, or add to food processor or high-speed blender and pulse until finely chopped, with some texture remaining. Sprinkle chopped almonds over clams.

9. Place in oven and bake about 10 minutes, until clams are just cooked through and topping is golden brown and aromatic.

10. Remove from oven and transfer to serving dish.

11. Serve immediately.

Jalapeño Lime Soft Pretzel

Prep Time: 15 minutes

Cook Time: 20 minutes

Servings: 4

INGREDIENTS

1 cup coconut flour

1/2 cup tapioca flour

1/2 cup coconut oil

1/2 cup water

1 egg

Juice of 1/2 lime

Zest if 1/2 lime

1 fresh jalapeño (or 2 oz pickled jalapeño)

2 tablespoons apple cider vinegar

1/2 teaspoon baking soda

1/2 teaspoon baking powder

1/2 teaspoon sea salt

Cilantro Lime Almond Cheese

1 cup soaked, skinless almonds*

3/4 cup water

1 tablespoons coconut oil

Juice of 1/2 lime

1 clove garlic

1/2 teaspoon sea salt

Pinch ground black pepper

Small bunch cilantro

1 1/2 cups water (for soaking)

INSTRUCTIONS

1. *Soak almonds in 1 1/2 cups water overnight. Drain and remove skins.
2. Preheat oven to 350 degrees F. Heat medium pot over medium-high heat. Line sheet pan with parchment or baking mat.
3. Add coconut oil, water, vinegar and salt to pot. Bring to a boil and remove from heat.
4. Whisk in tapioca flour. Stir with wooden spoon or soft spatula until mixture gels and comes together.
5. Stir in baking soda and baking powder. Mix for 1 minute. Mixture will foam and expand. Let mixture sit and cool about 5 minutes.
6. Remove stem, seed and veins from jalapeño and mince. Zest lime into pot, then add juice and jalapeño. Mix to incorporate.
7. Sift in coconut flour. Mix partially, then beat in egg. Blend until combined. Excess coconut flour may sit in bottom of bowl.
8. Turn out dough onto cutting board dusted with any excess coconut flour from mixture. Knead dough for 2 minutes.
9. Cut dough into 4 equal portions. Roll out pieces into ropes and twist to form classic pretzel twist. Pinch together any crumbled dough.
10. Arrange pretzels on lined sheet pan. Brush with coconut oil or full-fat coconut milk for glossy finish.

11. Place sheet pan in oven and bake about 25 minutes, until cooked through and golden.

12. For *Lime Almond Cheese*, peel garlic and add to food processor or high-speed blender with soaked almonds, coconut oil, lime juice, cilantro, salt and pepper. Process until smooth. Add water as necessary to reach desired consistency. You may process, let it rest, then process again to reach desired consistency.

13. Transfer *Cilantro Lime Almond Cheese* to serving dish.

14. Remove pretzels from oven and serve warm with *Cilantro Lime Almond Cheese*.

Bacon Quesadilla

Prep Time: 10 minutes

Cook Time: 20 minutes

Servings: 2

INGREDIENTS

Filling

8 - 12 strips nitrate-free bacon

Tortillas

2 tablespoons almond flour

1 1/2 tablespoons coconut flour

1/2 tablespoon flax meal (or ground chia seed)

1/4 cup water

2 eggs

2 tablespoons coconut oil

1/4 teaspoon baking powder

Coconut oil (for cooking)

Almond Cheese

1 cup skinless almonds*

1/4 cup water

2 tablespoons coconut oil

1 tablespoon lemon juice

1 tablespoon apple cider vinegar

1 garlic clove

1/2 teaspoon sea salt

1/4 teaspoon ground white pepper (or black pepper)

Avocado Cream

1 avocado

1/4 cup full-fat coconut cream

Small bunch cilantro

Juice of half lime

INSTRUCTIONS

1. *For *Almond Cheese*, soak almonds in 1 1/2 cups water overnight. Drain and rinse.

2. Add all *Almond Cheese* ingredients to food processor or bullet blender and process until smooth. Add a few extra tablespoons of water if necessary to achieve thick but smooth consistency. Set aside.

3. Preheat oven to 425 degrees F. Heat medium skillet over medium-high heat.

4. Chop bacon and sauté in skillet until crisp and cooked through, about 5 minutes. Remove bacon and set aside.

5. Reserve half of bacon grease. Add small amount of coconut oil to pan.

6. For *Tortillas*, whisk together eggs, coconut oil and 1/4 cup water in medium bowl. In a separate bowl, blend coconut flour, almond flour, flax or chia seed, and baking powder.

7. Whisk as you slowly pour dry into wet ingredients. If batter appears too thick to spread fairly thin in pan, add up to 4 tablespoons of water 1 tablespoon at a time.

8. Use ladle or dry measure cup to pour 1/2 of batter into hot oiled pan. Tilt pan in circular motion as you pour so batter spreads thinly.

9. Cook batter for about 2 minutes, or until slightly golden and firm. Flip tortilla with tongs or spatula and cook another 2 minutes. Remove and place on paper towel or parchment.

10. Add reserved bacon grease and small amount of coconut oil to pan. Cook remaining batter for 2 minutes on each side.

11. For *Avocado Cream*, slice avocado in half and pit. Scoop flesh into food processor with coconut cream, lime juice and cilantro. Process until smooth. Transfer to serving dish.

12. To assemble quesadilla, spread *Almond Cheese* over both tortillas. Sprinkle one tortilla with crisp bacon and top with other tortilla.

13. Place quesadilla on sheet pan or baking pan. Bake for 5 minutes.

14. Slice quesadilla with sharp knife or pizza cutter. Serve hot with *Avocado Cream*.

Chicken Taquitos

Prep Time: 10 minutes

Cook Time: 20 minutes

Servings: 4

INGREDIENTS

Tortillas

2 tablespoons almond flour

1 1/2 tablespoons coconut flour

1/2 tablespoon flax meal (or ground chia seed)

1/4 cup water

2 eggs

2 tablespoons coconut oil

1/4 teaspoon baking powder

Coconut oil (for cooking)

Almond Cheese

1 cup skinless almonds*

1/4 cup water

2 tablespoons coconut oil

1 tablespoon lemon juice

1 tablespoon apple cider vinegar

1 garlic clove

1/2 teaspoon sea salt

1/4 teaspoon ground white pepper (or black pepper)

Filling

8 oz chicken

1/2 teaspoon paprika

1/2 teaspoon ground cumin

Salsa

2 plum tomatoes

1/2 small white onion

Small bunch cilantro

1 jalapeño pepper

Squeeze of lime juice

1/2 teaspoon sea salt

INSTRUCTIONS

1. *For *Almond Cheese*, soak almonds in 1 1/2 cups water overnight. Drain and rinse.

2. Add all *Almond Cheese* ingredients to food processor or bullet blender and process until smooth. Add a few extra tablespoons of water if necessary to achieve thick but smooth consistency. Set aside.

3. Heat medium pan over medium-high heat and coat with coconut oil. Preheat oven to 400 degrees F.

4. Whisk together eggs, coconut oil and 1/4 cup water in medium bowl. In a separate bowl, blend coconut flour, almond flour, flax or chia seed, and baking powder.

5. Whisk as you slowly pour dry into wet ingredients. If batter appears too thick to spread fairly thin in pan, add up to 4 tablespoons of water 1 tablespoon at a time.

6. Use ladle or dry measure cup to pour 1/4 of batter into hot oiled pan. Tilt pan in circular motion as you pour so batter spreads thinly.

7. Cook batter for about 2 minutes or until slightly golden and firm. Flip tortilla with tongs or spatula and cook another 2 minutes. Remove and place on paper towel or parchment.

8. Cook remaining batter for 2 minutes on each side. Re-oil pan as necessary.

9. Add 1 tablespoon oil to hot pan.

10. Chop chicken and add to hot oiled pan with paprika and cumin. Sauté about 5 minutes, until golden brown and cooked through.

11. For *Salsa*, finely chop tomato, onion, jalapeño, cilantro and mix with squeeze of lime and salt in serving dish bowl.

12. Spread *Almond Cheese* on tortillas and Place sautéed chicken and salsa down center of each tortilla. Tightly roll each tortilla into long tube and place on sheet pan or baking pan. Pierce wit toothpick to keep roll tight if preferred.

13. Place in oven and bake about 5 - 7 minutes, until just heated through.

14. Remove and serve warm.

Awesome Healthy Pastries

Sweet Potato Pecan Chess Pie

Prep Time: 20 minutes

Cook Time: 25 minutes

Servings: 6

INGREDIENTS

Crust

2 cups almond flour

1 egg

2 tablespoons coconut oil

1 teaspoon ground cinnamon

1/4 teaspoon sea salt

Filling

1 cup full-fat coconut milk

1 cup organic canned yams

1 cup whole pecans

1/2 cup chopped pecans

1 cup dried pitted dates

1/2 cup sweetener*

2 eggs

2 egg yolks

2 tablespoons coconut oil

1 1/2 tablespoons arrowroot powder

2 teaspoons cinnamon

1 teaspoon vanilla

1/4 teaspoon nutmeg

INSTRUCTIONS

1. Preheat oven to 350 degrees F. Coat 6 mini pie pans with coconut oil. Bring small pot of water to boil, leaving room for dates.

2. Add dates to boiling water for about 5 minutes, until tender. Drain and set aside.

3. For *Crust*, blend almond flour, cinnamon and salt in small mixing bowl. Mix in oil and egg until dough forms.

4. Press dough into pie plates with hand or wooden spoon. Bake about 10 minutes, until golden. Remove pie shells from oven and set aside.

5. For *Filling*, process softened dates in food processor or bullet blender with 1/2 cup coconut milk until broken down.

6. Add date mixture to medium mixing bowl with remaining coconut milk, yams, sweetener, eggs, egg yolks, coconut oil, arrowroot powder, vanilla, cinnamon and nutmeg. Beat with hand mixer or whisk until combined and a bit lightened. Mix in chopped pecans.

7. Pour batter into mini pie crusts. Top with 1 cup whole pecans and bake for 20 - 25 minutes, until filling is set.

8. Remove pies and let cool about 20 minutes before serving warm. Or refrigerate and serve cold. Also great at room temperature.

*stevia, raw honey or agave nectar

NOTE: For large **Sweet Potato Pecan Chess Pie**, bake in 9-inch pie pan for 45 - 55 minutes, or until center is set.

Cocoa-nut Cake

Prep Time: 10 minutes

Cook Time: 25 minutes

Servings: 12

INGREDIENTS

Chocolate Coconut Cake

3/4 cup coconut flour

6 eggs

1 cup flaked or shredded coconut

1 cup unsweetened applesauce

1/2 cup coconut oil

1/2 cup coconut milk

1/2 cup sweetener*

1/2 cup dried pitted dates

1/3 cup cocoa powder

1 teaspoon vanilla

1 teaspoon baking soda

1 teaspoon baking powder

1/2 teaspoon sea salt

Chocolate Coconut Topping

Coconut cream (settled from 1 can full-fat coconut milk)

2 - 4 tablespoons sweetener*

2 tablespoons cocoa powder

1/2 teaspoon vanilla

1/2 cup flaked or shredded coconut

INSTRUCTIONS

1. Preheat oven to 325 degrees F. Line two round or square baking pans with parchment or lightly coat with coconut oil.
2. For *Chocolate Coconut Cake*, add dates, coconut milk, and half of eggs and oil to food processor or high-speed blender. Process until fairly smooth, about 1 - 2 minutes.
3. Pour date mixture into medium bowl. Add applesauce, sweetener, vanilla, and remaining eggs and oil. Beat with hand mixer or whisk until well combined.
4. Sift coconut flour, cocoa, salt, and baking soda and powder into wet ingredients. Blend until smooth. Stir in coconut.
5. Divide batter and pour into prepared baking pans and bake for about 25 minutes, or until golden and toothpick inserted into center comes out clean.
6. For *Chocolate Coconut Topping*, beat coconut cream in medium mixing bowl until slightly thickened. Add sweetener, vanilla and cocoa. Continue to beat until fully thickened and fluffy.
7. Remove cakes from oven and allow to cool. Place in refrigerator to speed cooling.
8. Frost cooled cakes and stack one on top of the other. Evenly sprinkle flaked coconut over top layer.
9. Slice and serve.

*stevia, raw honey, agave nectar or maple syrup

Chocolate Pecan Shortbread Cookies

Prep Time: 5 minutes

Cook Time: 20 minutes

Servings: 12

INGREDIENTS

1 1/2 cups almond flour

1 1/2 cup pecans

1/4 cup cocoa powder

1/4 cup coconut oil (or melted cacao butter)

1/4 cup sweetener*

1 teaspoons vanilla

1/4 teaspoon baking soda

1/2 teaspoon sea salt

INSTRUCTIONS

1. Preheat oven to 300 degrees F. Line sheet pan with parchment or baking mat.
2. Add 1 cup pecans to food processor or high-speed blender and process until finely ground.
3. Add ground pecans to medium mixing bowl. Sift in almond flour, cocoa, baking soda and salt.
4. Chop remaining pecans and add to small mixing bowl. Add coconut oil or melted cacao butter, sweetener and vanilla to pecans. Mix to combine.
5. Pour wet mixture into dry ingredients and mix to form dough.

6. Use mini ice cream scoop or tablespoon to drop portions of dough onto prepared sheet pan.

7. Place in oven and bake 20 minutes, or until lightly browned.

8. Remove from oven and let cool at least 5 minutes.

9. Let cool completely and serve room temperature. Or serve warm.

*raw honey, agave nectar or maple syrup

Peach Pecan "Fried" Pie

Prep Time: 20 minutes

Cook Time: 20 minutes

Servings: 4

INSTRUCTIONS

Crust

2 cups almond flour

2 eggs

3 tablespoons coconut oil

1 tablespoon sweetener*

1/4 teaspoon baking soda

1 teaspoon ground cinnamon

1/2 teaspoon sea salt

Filling

2 peaches

1/4 cup dried apricots

1/4 cup pecans

2 tablespoons sweetener*

2 tablespoons water

1 tablespoon ground cinnamon

1 teaspoon vanilla

1/2 teaspoon ground ginger

DIRECTIONS

1. Preheat oven to 400 degrees. Line sheet pan with parchment or baking mat. Cover cutting board with parchment.
2. For *Crust*, sift almond flour into medium mixing bowl. Add baking soda, cinnamon and salt.
3. Whisk eggs and sweetener in small mixing bowl, then add to flour and combine. Slowly add coconut oil until malleable dough comes together.
4. Roll in plastic wrap or wrap tightly in parchment and refrigerate for 15 minutes.
5. Heat medium pan over medium heat.
6. Peel and pit peaches. Chop apricots, pecans and peaches. Add to hot pan with sweetener, spices and water. Sauté about 5 - 10 minutes, until peaches are tender and
7. Remove dough from refrigerator. Roll dough out on parchment covered cutting board to about 1/8 inch thick square with rolling pin. Use sharp knife or pizza cutter to cut dough into 4 squares.
8. Scoop equal portions of *Filling* into center of one side of each dough square. Fold bare half of dough over filled half. Press edges together, letting any trapped air escape. Crimp edges of dough together with fork. Repeat with remaining dough.
9. Arrange pies on lined sheet pan and bake 15 - 20 minutes, or until dough is golden and cooked through.
10. Serve immediately. Or allow to cool and store in air-tight container.

*stevia, raw honey or agave nectar

NOTE: Heat large skillet over medium heat , add 1/4 inch coconut oil, and fry pies 2 minutes on each side for traditional *Fried Pies*.

Sweet Potato "Fried" Pie

Prep Time: 20 minutes

Cook Time: 30 minutes

Servings: 4

INSTRUCTIONS

Crust

2 cups almond flour

2 eggs

3 tablespoons coconut oil

1 tablespoon sweetener*

1/4 teaspoon baking soda

1/2 teaspoon ground cinnamon

1/2 teaspoon sea salt

Filling

1 large sweet potato

1/2 cup dried dates

1/4 cup walnuts

1 egg

1 teaspoon vanilla

1 teaspoon ground cinnamon

1 teaspoon ground nutmeg

1/2 teaspoon ground black pepper

DIRECTIONS

1. Bring medium pot of lightly salted water to boil. Cover cutting board with parchment.

2. For *Crust*, sift almond flour into medium mixing bowl. Add baking soda, cinnamon and salt.

3. Whisk eggs and sweetener in small mixing bowl, then add to flour and combine. Slowly add coconut oil until malleable dough comes together.

4. Roll in plastic wrap or wrap tightly in parchment and refrigerate for 15 minutes.

5. Preheat oven to 400 degrees. Line sheet pan with parchment or baking mat.

6. Peel and dice sweet potato. Chop dates. Add sweet potato and dates to boiling water peaches. Cook about 10 minutes, until sweet potatoes are soft. Drain sweet potatoes and dates.

7. Add egg to medium mixing bowl. Add 1 tablespoon hot sweet potatoes to bowl. Mash briefly, then add second tablespoon. Gradually add all hot sweet potatoes and dates to egg. Mash and mix, careful not to scramble egg. Stir in vanilla, cinnamon, nutmeg and pepper.

8. Chop walnuts. Set aside.

9. Remove dough from refrigerator. Roll dough out on parchment covered cutting board to about 1/8 inch thick square with rolling pin. Use sharp knife or pizza cutter to cut dough into 4 squares.

10. Scoop equal portions of *Filling* into center of one side of each dough square. Fold bare half of dough over filled half. Press

edges together, letting any trapped air escape. Crimp edges of dough together with fork. Repeat with remaining dough.

11. Arrange pies on lined sheet pan and bake 15 - 20 minutes, or until dough is golden and cooked through.

12. Serve immediately. Or allow to cool and store in air-tight container.

stevia, raw honey or agave nectar

NOTE: Heat large skillet over medium heat , add 1/4 inch coconut oil, and fry pies 2 minutes on each side for traditional *Fried Pies*.

Sugar-Free Coconut Cake

Prep Time: 10 minutes

Cook Time: 25 minutes

Servings: 12

INGREDIENTS

Coconut Cake

6 cage-free eggs

3/4 cup coconut flour

1 cup flaked coconut

1 cup unsweetened applesauce

1/2 cup coconut oil

1/2 cup coconut milk

1/2 cup sweetener*

1/2 cup dried pitted dates

2 teaspoons vanilla

1 teaspoon baking soda

1 teaspoon baking powder

1/2 teaspoon sea salt

Coconut Frosting

1/3 cup coconut cream (from 1 can settled full-fat coconut milk)

2 - 4 tablespoons sweetener*

1/2 teaspoon vanilla

1/2 cup flaked coconut

INSTRUCTIONS

1. Preheat oven to 325°F. Line two or square baking pans with parchment or coat lightly with coconut oil.

2. Add dates, coconut milk, and half of eggs and oil to food processor or bullet blender. Process until dates a broken down, about 1 - 2 minutes.

3. Pour date mixture into medium bowl. Add applesauce, sweetener, vanilla, and remaining eggs and oil. Beat with hand mixer or whisk until well combined.

4. Sift coconut flour, salt, and baking soda and baking powder into wet ingredients. Blend until smooth. Stir in coconut.

5. Pour batter into prepared baking pans and bake for about 25 minutes, or until golden and toothpick inserted into center comes out clean.

6. Remove from oven and allow to cool. Place in refrigerator to speed cooling.

7. For *Coconut Frosting*, beat coconut cream in medium mixing bowl until slightly thickened. Add sweetener and vanilla, and continue to beat until full thickened and fluffy.

8. Frost cooled cakes and stack one on top of the other. Evenly sprinkle flaked coconut on top layer of frosted cake.

9. Slice and serve.

*stevia, raw honey, agave nectar or maple syrup

Coconut Cream Pie

Prep Time: 20 minutes*

Cook Time: 20 minutes

Servings: 8

INGREDIENTS

Crust

1/2 cup soft nuts**

1 cup almond flour

2 teaspoons sweetener***

1/4 - 1/2 cup coconut oil

Filling

26 oz (2 cans) full-fat coconut milk

2 eggs

1/2 cup arrowroot powder

1/4 cup sweetener*

1 tablespoon vanilla

1 cup flaked coconut

Pinch sea salt

INSTRUCTIONS

1. Preheat oven to 350 degrees F. Lightly coast pie plate with coconut oil.

2. Grind nuts into coarse meal with food processor or bullet blender. Add to small bowl with almond flour, 2 tablespoons

sweetener and enough coconut oil to bring together soft but crumbly dough.

3. Press dough into pie plate and bake about 10 - 15 minutes, until crust becomes golden.

4. Remove crust from oven and allow to cool. Turn off oven.

5. Add coconut milk, eggs, arrowroot powder, sweetener, vanilla and salt to medium pot. Heat pot over medium heat and bring to a boil. Stir constantly as mixture thickens.

6. Stir in 1/2 cup shredded coconut. Then pour the filling over the crust.

7. *Refrigerate pie until filling is set, about 4 hours.

8. Heat medium pan over medium heat. Add 1/2 cup flaked coconut and toast about 5 minutes. Stir frequently to prevent burning.

9. Sprinkle toasted coconut over pie and serve chilled.

NOTE: Line springform pan with parchment and bake crust, then fill with coconut cream filling for another version of **Coconut Cream Pie**.

**coconut flakes, pecans, walnuts, cashews or brazil nuts
***stevia, raw honey or agave nectar

Wild Mince Meat Pie

Prep Time: 20 minutes

Cook Time: 30 minutes

Servings: 8

INGREDIENTS

Crust

4 cups almond flour

2 eggs

1/4 cup coconut oil

1/2 teaspoon sea salt

Filling

12 oz grass-fed beef

2 sweet apples

2 tart apples

1 cup beef stock

1/4 cup sweetener*

Juice of 1 orange

Zest of 1 orange

1/4 cup arrowroot powder

1/4 cup apple cider vinegar

1 cup raisins

1/2 cup dried pitted dates

1/2 cup dried pitted prunes

1/2 cup dried cherries

2 teaspoons ground cinnamon

1 teaspoon ground nutmeg

1/2 teaspoon ground cloves

1/2 teaspoon ground black pepper

1/2 teaspoon salt

INSTRUCTIONS

1. Preheat oven to 350 degrees F. Heat large pot over medium-high heat and lightly coat with coconut oil. Lightly oil pie plate. Prepare 4 sheets of parchment.

2. Place beef in hot oiled pan and brown on each side for about 5 - 7 minutes, until just cooked through. Remove beef and set aside. Add beef stock to pot.

3. Mix all *Crust* ingredients together in medium bowl until dough forms. Divide dough in half and use rolling pin to roll dough between two parchment sheets into circles to fit about 1 inch over pie plate.

4. Press one dough circle into pie plate. Crimp edges to create small lip. Bake for 5 minutes, then remove and set aside.

5. Peel, core and grate or dice apples. Add to beef stock with sweetener, zest and juice of orange, vinegar, raisins, cherries, spices and salt. Dice beef, prunes and dates, and add to pot. Stir in arrowroot powder and thicken for a few minutes.

6. Once mixture comes together pour into par baked pie shell. Top with second dough sheet and crimp edges to fit into bottom crust.

7. Use sharp knife to slice top crust a few times for venting.

8. Bake pie for 30 minutes, or until crust is golden brown.

9. Remove from oven and allow to cool for about 20 minutes.

10. Slice and serve warm. Or allow to cool completely and serve room temperature.

stevia, raw honey or agave nectar

Chocolate Almond Biscotti

Prep Time: 15 minutes

Cook Time: 35* minutes

Servings: 6

INGREDIENTS

1 cup almond flour

1/2 cup coconut flour

1/2 cup sweetener*

1/3 cup almonds

2 tablespoons cocoa powder

1 teaspoon vanilla

1/2 teaspoon baking soda

1/4 teaspoon sea salt

INSTRUCTIONS

1. Preheat oven to 350 degrees F. Line sheet pan with parchment paper. Heat medium pan over medium heat.

2. Add almonds to hot dry pan and toast for about 5 minutes, until aromatic. Stir frequently. Remove from heat and set aside.

3. In medium mixing bowl, blend almond flour, coconut flour, cocoa powder, baking soda and salt with hand mixer or whisk.

4. Beat in sweetener and vanilla until well combined and thick, sticky dough forms. Mix in toasted almonds with wooden spoon.

5. Form dough into flattened, uniform mound about 1 inch thick on sheet pan. Pat down mound to keep any almonds from sticking out.

6. Bake for about 15 minutes . Remove and allow to cool for about 15 minutes.

7. Use a very sharp serrated knife to carefully cut biscotti log into 1/2 - 2/3 inch slices. Hold onto the mound and cut on a diagonal. If it becomes crumbly, stick it back together.

8. Lace slice on sides and return to oven for 15 minutes.

9. Try to cut so that you're holding on to the edges of the log to keep it from crumbling. If parts come apart, you can stick them back together as the mixture is still kind of sticky.

10. Lay the biscotti flat and return to oven for 15 minutes.

11. *Turn oven off and leave oven door open a crack. Allow the biscotti to cool and dry for at least 2 hours.

12. Serve room temperature.

*raw honey, agave nectar, maple syrup, or any combination

Crab Boil Biscuits

Prep Time: 5 minutes

Cook Time: 15 minutes

Servings: 12

INGREDIENTS

1 cup almond flour

6 oz (1 can) lump crab meat

2 eggs

1/4 cup coconut oil

1 tablespoon apple cider vinegar

1 1/2 teaspoons baking powder

2 teaspoons crab boil spice blend

1/2 teaspoon ground black pepper

1/2 teaspoon ground turmeric (optional)

1/4 teaspoon Sea salt

INSTRUCTIONS

1. Preheat oven to 350 degrees F. Line muffin pan with paper liners or lightly coat with coconut oil. Or cover sheet pan with parchment or baking mat.

2. Beat eggs in medium mixing bowl with hand mixer or whisk until thick and slightly frothy. Add drained lump crab meat, coconut oil and vinegar. Mix well.

3. Stir in almond flour, baking powder, salt and spices until combined.

4. Use ice cream scoop or tablespoon to scoop batter onto prepare muffin pan or sheet pan.
5. Place in oven and bake 15 - 18 minutes, until edges are golden brown and tops are firm.
6. Remove from oven and let cool slightly.
7. Serve warm. Or allow to cool completely and serve room temperature.

Crispy Almond Pizza Crust

Prep Time: 5 minutes

Cook Time: 10 minutes

Servings: 2

INGREDIENTS

1 cup almond flour

1 Egg

1/2 tablespoon coconut oil

1/2 teaspoon sea salt

Pinch ground black pepper

Extra almond flour

Coconut oil (for baking)

Optional Spices:

1 teaspoon dried basil

DIRECTIONS

1. Preheat oven to 350 degrees F. Cover sheet pan with parchment paper or baking mat, or coat with coconut oil. Prepare two additional sheets of parchment and set aside on cutting board.

2. Combine all ingredients, plus *Optional Spices*, in small bowl. If too soft, add 1 tablespoon of almond flour at a time until firm dough that can hold its shape forms.

3. Form dough into ball and place on parchment covered cutting board. Press dough with palms to flatten. Then cover dough with parchment sheet and roll thin with rolling pin.

4. Carefully remove top layer of parchment from flattened dough, and place fresh parchment sheet over crust. Place sheet pan upside down over crust and careful flip thin crust onto sheet pan. Use cutting board for support to keep crust intact. Carefully peel off parchment layer (that was on the bottom and is now on top).

5. Bake crust on sheet pan in preheated oven for 5 minutes.

6. Carefully remove par baked crust and evenly spread and sprinkle with favorite sauce and toppings.

7. Return pizza to oven and bake another 5 - 10 minutes, or until toppings are heated through. Take care not to burn thin crust.

8. Turn off oven. Slice and serve hot.

9. Leave leftovers directly on oven rack (no sheet pan) to keep crust crispy.

Chewy Coconut Pizza Dough

Prep Time: 5 minutes

Cook Time: 20 minutes

Servings: 2

INGREDIENTS

1/3 cup coconut flour

1/4 cup flax meal (or ground chia seed)

3 Eggs

1/2 cup coconut milk

1/2 teaspoon salt

1 teaspoon baking powder

Optional Spices:

1 teaspoon dried oregano

1/2 teaspoon ground basil

INSTRUCTIONS

1. Preheat oven to 350 degrees F. Cover sheet pan with parchment paper, baking mat, or aluminum foil coated with coconut oil. Prepare additional sheet of parchment or aluminum (optional).
2. In medium bowl, beat eggs with coconut milk with hand mixer or whisk. Sift in coconut flour, flax, salt, baking powder and *Optional Spices*. Beat into thick batter.
3. Spread batter in desired shape on sheet pan with ladle or spatula.

4. Bake for 10 minutes or until firm enough to flip.

5. Carefully remove par baked crust. Peel away from sheet pan and flip. Or flip parchment or aluminum sheet and crust onto fresh sheet. Then peel crust away from used parchment or aluminum sheet.

6. Return crust to oven and bake for additional 8 - 10 minutes, or until cooked through.

7. Remove crust again, and evenly spread and sprinkle with favorite sauce and toppings.

8. Set oven to broil and broil pizza for 1 - 2 minutes, just to heat toppings.

9. Remove pizza . Slice with knife or pizza cutter and serve hot.

Cashew Belgian Waffles

Prep Time: 10 minutes

Cook Time: 10 minutes

Servings: 2

INGREDIENTS

Waffles:

1 cup cashew flour (or finely ground raw cashews)

1/4 coconut flour

3 eggs, separated

1/4 cup coconut oil

4 tablespoons sweetener

1 tablespoon aluminum-free baking soda

1 teaspoon vanilla

1 pinch sea salt

1 teaspoon ground cinnamon (optional)

Topping:

1 cup fresh fruit

1/2 teaspoon vanilla

2 tablespoons water

1 tablespoon sweetener*

DIRECTIONS

1. Preheat waffle iron. Use wadded paper towel to carefully coat with coconut oil.

2. Combine flours, salt and baking soda in small bowl. In large bowl, whisk together egg yolks, oil, vanilla, plus sweetener and cinnamon (optional).
3. In separate bowl, beat egg whites to medium-stiff peaks with hand mixer. Stir flour mixture into the egg yolk mixture. Gently fold egg whites into batter.
4. Pour portion of batter onto hot waffle iron. Cook 4 - 5 minutes, until golden brown and crisp. Repeat with remain batter
5. While waffles are cooking, combine all **Topping** ingredients in small pan. Cook over stovetop until reduced and thick.
6. Top waffles with fruit compote or agave syrup (optional). Serve hot.

stevia, raw honey, or agave nectar

Double Pumpkin Muffins

Prep Time: 5 minutes

Cook Time: 25 minutes

Servings: 12

INGREDIENTS

1 3/4 cups coconut flour

2 cage-free eggs

15 oz (1 can) organic pumpkin puree

1 cup unsweetened applesauce

1/2 cup coconut oil

1/4 cup sweetener*

2 teaspoons baking soda

1 1/2 tablespoon ground cinnamon

1/2 teaspoon ground nutmeg

1 teaspoon sea salt

1/2 cup pumpkin seeds

INSTRUCTIONS

1. Preheat oven to 350 degrees F. Line muffin pan with paper liner or coat with coconut oil.
2. Process eggs, coconut oil, applesauce and sweetener in food processor or blender until thick and light, about 2 minutes.
3. Pour egg mixture into medium mixing bowl. Add pumpkin puree, salt and spices and mix with hand mixer or whisk.

4. Sift in coconut flour and baking soda. Mix until well combined. Stir in half of pumpkin seeds.

5. Pour batter into prepared muffin pan and sprinkle remaining pumpkin seeds over batter.

6. Place in oven and bake 20 - 25 minutes , until edges are golden and tops firm but springy.

7. Remove from oven and allow to cool 5 minutes.

8. Serve warm. Or let cool complete and serve room temperature.

*stevia, raw honey or agave nectar

Classic Bagels

Prep Time: 10 minutes

Cook Time: 25 minutes

Servings: 8

INGREDIENTS

2 cups almond flour

2 tablespoons coconut flour

2 tablespoons ground chia seed (or flax meal)

1 tablespoon tapioca flour (or arrowroot powder)

4 cage-free eggs

1/3 cup apple cider vinegar

2 tablespoons unsweetened applesauce

2 tablespoons sweetener*

1 teaspoon baking soda

1/2 teaspoon sea salt

INSTRUCTIONS

1. Preheat oven to 350 degrees. Lightly coat donut pan with coconut oil.

2. Add almond, coconut and tapioca flours, chia meal, baking soda and salt to food processor or bullet blender, and process for 1 minute.

3. Add eggs, sweetener, applesauce and apple cider vinegar to flour mixture and process until fully blended, about 1 - 2 minutes.

4. Carefully scoop batter into donut pan, avoiding raised middle.
5. Place in oven and bake about 20 - 25 minutes.
6. Remove and let cool about 5 minutes. Then remove from pan.
7. Slice in half and serve immediately. Or let cool completely and serve room temperature.

NOTE: Bake in 8 round mini cake pans lightly coated with coconut oil if you do not have a donut pan.

stevia, raw honey or agave nectar

Plain Pita

Prep Time: 5 minutes

Cook Time: 20 minutes

Servings: 1

INGREDIENTS

1 cup tapioca flour

1 cage-free egg

1/4 cup water

2 tablespoons coconut oil

1 teaspoon ground chia seed (or flax meal)

1/2 teaspoon baking soda

1/4 teaspoon ground white pepper (or black pepper)

1/4 teaspoon sea salt

INSTRUCTIONS

1. Preheat the oven to 375 degrees F. Line sheet pan with parchment paper or baking mat, or lightly coat with coconut oil. Heat small pot over low heat.

2. Add 1/3 cup tapioca flour, chia meal, water and 1 tablespoon coconut oil to pot. Stir until mixture comes together. Remove from heat and cool in freezer.

3. In medium bowl, blend remaining tapioca flour, baking soda, salt and pepper. Then add egg and remaining oil. Mix until combined.

4. Add cooled chia mixture to bowl. Mix to combine, then remove and knead briefly to bring together dough.

5. Form round disk, then flatten on prepared sheet pan to 1/4 - 1/3 inch with hands or rolling pin.

6. Place in oven and bake about 15 minutes. Carefully remove pan and turn pita over with spatula. Return to oven and bake another 5 - 10 minutes, or until crisp.

7. Remove from oven and fill with favorite Mediterranean meats. Or cut into wedges and dip into favorite spreads.

8. Serve warm or room temperature.

Sesame Pretzel Sticks

Prep Time: 15 minutes

Cook Time: 20 minutes

Servings: 6

INGREDIENTS

1 cup coconut flour

1/2 cup tapioca flour

1/3 cup coconut oil

2 tablespoons unsweetened applesauce

1/2 cup water

1 cage-free egg

2 tablespoons apple cider vinegar

1/2 teaspoon baking soda

1/2 teaspoon baking powder

1/2 teaspoon sea salt

1 tablespoon sesame seeds

INSTRUCTIONS

1. Preheat oven to 350 degrees F. Heat medium pan over medium-high heat. Line sheet pan with parchment or baking mat.
2. Add coconut oil, water, vinegar and salt to pot. Bring to a boil and remove from heat. Stir in apple sauce.
3. Whisk in tapioca flour. Stir with wooden spoon or soft spatula until mixture gels and comes together.

4. Stir in baking soda and baking powder. Continue mixing for about 1 minute. Mixture will foam and expand. Let mixture sit and cool about 5 minutes.

5. Sift in coconut flour. Mix partially, then beat in egg. Blend until combined. Excess coconut flour may sit in bottom of bowl.

6. Turn out dough onto cutting board dusted with any excess coconut flour from mixture. Knead dough for 2 minutes.

7. Cut dough into 6 equal portions. Roll out pieces into ropes, then lay straight on prepared sheet pan. Use knife to score dough diagonally a few times for presentation.

8. Brush with coconut oil or full-fat coconut milk and sprinkle with sesame seeds.

9. Place sheet pan in oven and bake about 20 - 25 minutes, until cooked through.

10. Serve immediately with favorite dipping sauce. Or allow to cool and serve room temperature.

Chicken Dumpling Bun

Prep Time: 15 minutes

Cook Time: 20 minutes

Servings: 4

INGREDIENTS

Dumpling Bun

1 cup tapioca flour

1/4 - 1/3 cup coconut flour

1 cage-free egg

1/2 cup warm chicken stock

1/4 cup coconut oil

1/4 cup applesauce

1 teaspoon apple cider vinegar

1 teaspoon baking soda

1/2 teaspoon onion powder

1/ 4 teaspoon garlic powder

1/2 teaspoon sea salt

Filling

8 oz boneless chicken (breasts, thighs, etc.)

1 small carrot

1 small celery stalk

1/2 teaspoon dried thyme

1/4 teaspoon ground sage

1/2 teaspoon ground black pepper

1/2 teaspoon sea salt

INSTRUCTIONS

1. Preheat oven to 350 degrees F. Line sheet pan with parchment paper or coat with coconut oil. Heat medium skillet over medium heat and lightly coat with coconut oil.
2. Add chicken stock to small pot and heat over medium heat.
3. For *Filling*, dice carrot and celery, fillet chicken in half, and add to hot oiled skillet with salt and spices. Sauté until chicken is cooked through and browned and veggies are softened, about 5 - 8 minutes. Remove from heat and set aside. Shred or dice rested chicken and mix thoroughly with sautéed veggies.
4. For *Dumpling Bun*, sift together tapioca flour, coconut flour, baking soda, salt and spices in medium bowl.
5. Whisk egg, applesauce and vinegar in small bowl. Whisk in warm chicken stock and coconut oil.
6. Add egg mixture to flour mixture and mix until well combined. Add 1 tablespoon coconut flour or water at a time if needed to form soft and slightly sticky dough.
7. Divide dough into 4 portions and flatten into round disks. Dust your hand or rolling pin with extra tapioca flour to prevent sticking.
8. Scoop chicken *Filling* into center of each dough disk and pinch edges of dough together to create round, sealed ball.
9. Place filled buns sealed side down on sheet pan and pat down slightly.

10. Place in oven and bake 20 minutes, or until edges are golden brown and dough is cooked through.
11. Remove from oven and let cool about 5 minutes.
12. Serve warm.

Sweet Potato Cinnamon Rolls

Prep Time: 10 minutes

Cook Time: 20 minutes

Servings: 8

INGREDIENTS

Sweet Potato Roll

1 cup tapioca flour

1/4 - 1/3 cup coconut flour

1 cage-free egg

1/2 cup organic canned yams

1/4 cup warm water

1/4 cup coconut oil

1 - 2 tablespoons sweetener*

1 teaspoon apple cider vinegar

1 teaspoon baking soda

1/2 teaspoon ground cinnamon

1/2 teaspoon nutmeg

1/4 teaspoon ground black pepper

1 teaspoon sea salt

Cinnamon Swirl

4 - 5 dried pitted dates

1 teaspoon tapioca flour

1 tablespoon ground cinnamon

1/4 cup hot water

INSTRUCTIONS

1. Preheat oven to 350 degrees F. Line muffin pan with paper liners or coat with coconut oil. Heat water in small pan over medium heat. Cover cutting board with parchment.

2. For *Cinnamon Swirl*, add dates, tapioca, cinnamon, and hot water to food processor or bullet blender. Process until dates are broken down and thick mixture forms. Set aside.

3. For *Sweet Potato Roll*, sift tapioca flour, 1/4 cup coconut flour, baking soda, salt and spices into In medium bowl.

4. In small bowl, beat egg, yams, sweetener and vinegar with hand mixer or whisk until well combined. Beat in warm water and oil.

5. Add yam mixture to dry ingredients and mix until well combined. If necessary, add coconut flour or water 1 tablespoon at a time to form a soft and slightly sticky dough.

6. Dust parchment covered cutting board and hands with tapioca flour to prevent sticking. Turn dough out onto parchment. Use dusted hands or rolling pin to flatten dough into 1/2 inch thick square.

7. Use spoon or knife to spread *Cinnamon Swirl* evenly over dough. Roll dough into log and cut into 8 slices, approximately 1 - 1 1/2 inch thick.

8. Turn rolls swirl side up and place in prepared muffin pan.

9. Place in oven and bake about 20 minutes, or until edges browned, cinnamon bubbles, and tops are firm.

10. Remove from oven and let cool about 5 minutes.

11. Serve immediately. Or let cool and serve or room temperature or chilled.

stevia, raw honey or agave nectar

Pumpkin Spice Cakes

Prep Time: 5 minutes

Cook Time: 15 minutes

Servings: 12

INGREDIENTS

3/4 cup coconut flour

4 eggs

1/4 cup coconut oil

1/2 cup sweetener*

1/2 cup pumpkin purée

1 teaspoon baking soda

1 tablespoon ground cinnamon

1 tablespoon ground ginger

1 tablespoon ground nutmeg

1 tablespoon ground black pepper

1 teaspoon vanilla

1/2 teaspoon sea salt

1/4 cup pumpkin seeds

INSTRUCTIONS

1. Preheat oven to 350 degrees F. Lightly coat 4 mini cake pans or mini loaf pans with coconut oil, or line with parchment paper.
2. Sift coconut flour, baking soda, salt and spices into large mixing bowl.

3. In medium mixing bowl, beat egg whites to soft peaks with hand mixer or whisk. About 5 minutes.

4. Then beat in yolks, oil, sweetener and pumpkin purée. Mix wet ingredients into dry blend until combined.

5. Pour batter into mini cake loaf pans and sprinkle on pumpkin seeds.

6. Bake for 20 - 25 minutes, or until firm but springy in the center and browned. A toothpick inserted into the middle should come out clean.

7. Remove from oven and allow to cool for 5 minutes before serving.

8. Serve warm or room temperature.

NOTE: For large **Pumpkin Spice Cake**, oil large loaf pan or springform pan and bake 40 - 45 minutes.

raw honey, agave nectar or maple syrup

Fruit And Nut Cake

Prep Time: 10 minutes

Cook Time: 25 minutes

Servings: 8

INGREDIENTS

1 1/2 cup almond flour

4 eggs

2 tablespoons coconut oil

Juice of orange half

1/4 cup sweetener*

1/2 cup walnuts

1/4 cup pecans

1/2 cup dried pitted dates

1/2 cup dried cherries

1/4 cup dried apricots

1/4 cup raisins

1/2 teaspoon baking soda

1 teaspoon ground ginger

1 teaspoon vanilla

1/2 teaspoon sea salt

Zest of orange half

INSTRUCTIONS

1. Preheat oven to 350 degrees F. Lightly coat 2 small loaf pans or one Bundt pan with coconut oil.

2. Sift almond flour, baking soda and salt into large mixing bowl.

3. Chop walnuts, pecans, apricots and dates. Then stir all dried fruit and nuts into flour mixture.

4. In medium mixing bowl, mix eggs, coconut oil, juice and zest of half an orange, sweetener, ginger and vanilla. Then pour and mix into dry ingredients until just combined.

5. Scoop batter into loaf pans or Bundt pan, and smooth tops with spatula.

6. Bake 20 - 30 minutes, or until firm, browned and firm in the center.

7. Remove from oven and allow to cool before slicing.

8. Serve warm or room temperature.

*stevia, raw honey or agave nectar

Toasted Almond Cream Cakes

Prep Time: 15 minutes*

Cook Time: 20 minutes

Servings: 12

INGREDIENTS

Cake

1 cup almond flour

4 egg whites

1/3 cup coconut oil

1/4 cup almond milk

1/4 cup sweetener*

1 teaspoon baking powder

1/4 cup slice almonds

Almond Cream

2 cups skinless almonds

1/4 cup sweetener

1 teaspoon vanilla

Water

INSTRUCTIONS

1. *Soak almonds overnight in water. Drain and rinse.
2. Preheat the oven to 350 degrees F. Heat medium pan over medium heat. Lightly coat muffin pan with coconut oil, or line with paper liners

3. Add almond flour to hot dry pan and toast about 5 minutes, stirring frequently. Do not burn. Remove from heat and set aside.

4. Beat egg whites to soft peaks with hand mixer or whisk in medium bowl. Then beat in oil, milk and 1/4 cup sweetener. Sift in toasted almond flour and baking powder. Mix until just combined.

5. Use ice cream scoop or spoon to scoop batter into muffin pan. Each cup should be only 1/2 full.

6. Bake about 15 minutes, or until center is set but springy.

7. Remove pan from oven and remove cakes from pan. Let cool for about 15 minutes.

8. While cakes cool, blend soaked almonds, 1/4 cup sweetener, 1 teaspoon vanilla and water as needed in food processor or blender to make smooth *Almond Cream*.

9. Wipe out pan with paper towel and return dry pan to medium heat. Toast slice almonds about 5 minutes, until aromatic and golden. Do not burn. Remove from heat and set aside.

10. When cakes are cooled, slice in half to create top and bottom layer. Scoop cream onto bottom half, and top with top half of cake. Scoop another dollop of cream over top half and sprinkle on slice toasted almonds.

11. Serve room temperature.

NOTE: For large **Toasted Almond Cream Cake** , bake batter in 2 round cake pans for 35 - 40 minutes.

raw honey, agave nectar or maple syrup

www.ingramcontent.com/pod-product-compliance
Lightning Source LLC
Chambersburg PA
CBHW071359310526
45790CB00019B/1447